HY[illegible]
ACUPUNCTURE
AND PAIN

Alternative Methods for Treatment

by

Maurice M. Tinterow, M.D., Ph.D.

Bio-Communications Press
3100 North Hillside
Wichita, Kansas 67219

For information address:

BIO-COMMUNICATIONS PRESS
3100 North Hillside Avenue
Wichita, Kansas 67219 USA

ISBN 0-942333-08-X
Library of Congress Catalog Card Number: 89-62007

First Edition

Published in the United States of America

DEDICATION

To Dr. Hugh Riordan, who does not see aging as a termination to a career and who welcomed the opportunity for me to continue the art of hypnotherapy and acupuncture in the practice of holistic medicine.

Maurice M. Tinterow, M.D., Ph.D.

TABLE OF CONTENTS

FOREWORD

Pain and suffering is a problem as old as mankind. A whole multitude of explanations have been offered over time attempting to make sense of the fact that all people, sooner or later, suffer pain. Philosophers, theologians, social scientists and many others have sought lofty understandings.

The clinician experiences pain from another perspective. Clinicians have taken oaths to help alleviate pain wherever possible. The clinician is less interested in lofty explanations, and rather seeks in its place practical interventions for pain.

Modern medical technology has delivered many new tools to assist the clinician in the alleviation of pain. In spite of advances, pain remains a perennial problem which still eludes the clinical practitioner from possessing absolute solutions.

Ironically, some of the more potent treatments for pain turn out to be some of our older treatments. Persons who have not responded well to modern chemical analgesics have found themselves in recent years resorting successfully to alternative therapies—which in fact turn out to be not "new" but "old" therapies.

Two of the best alternative treatments for pain are hypnosis and acupuncture. Unfortunately both of these treatments have experienced a great deal of derision, attack and misunderstanding over time.

Dr. Maurice Tinterow has trained extensively in both treatment modalities. As an anesthesiologist, his many years of experience of integrating hypnosis and acupuncture into the treatment of pain—both in anesthesia for surgery, and also with chronic problems in a pain clinic—qualifies him as a unique teacher in this area.

This book helps to demystify much of the confusion that has surrounded these two treatment modalities, and enlightens the health practitioner regarding the values of their use in modern clinical practice.

Dr. Tinterow, author of a classic and authoritative work on the history of hypnosis, Foundations of Hypnosis (Tinterow, 1970), has given us another valuable book which is right for our times.

Jon M. Sward, J.D., Ph.D.—June, 1989

References

Tinterow, M. M. (1970). Foundations of Hypnosis. Springfield, Ill.: C. C. Thomas.

PREFACE

I am in my third career, having been an anesthesiologist for forty years, an educator for six years and I am now practising in the field of holistic medicine. Since anesthesia may be defined as the loss of sensation with or without the loss of consciousness that may be caused by disease, injury, chemical agents or psychological means, hypnosis can play a great part in relieving the discomfort and pain of the patient. My interest in using hypnosis as an integral part in treating pain led me to study the subject in great depth. The more I became involved, the more I could see the benefits of hypnosis. I started to read the history of Mesmerism, Animal Magnetism and Hypnosis, and collected 640 rare books, including nearly all of Mesmer and Braid. I donated that collection of books to the Rare Book Collection Department of the Wichita State University as The Maurice M. and Jean H. Tinterow Rare Book Collection. It is available for all those interested in the history of hypnosis to read and review, since it is as complete a collection as there is in the United States.

There were those who could not be anesthetized in the usual manner with drugs and anesthetic agents. Reading Esdaile's book on the use of Mesmeric anesthesia in India, in which he performed many operations using Mesmerism, since chemical anesthetics had not yet become a part of the practice of medicine, I was sure that surgical procedures could be performed under hypnotic anesthesia. The first operative procedure in 1960, performed under hypnotic anesthesia was a vaginal hysterectomy, and I was surprised at the decrease in the loss of blood in a patient who was relaxed. I have done many more operative procedures with success, and I am of the opinion that it should be used more by anesthesiologists for those procedures in which there is contraindication to the use of usual narcotic and chemical agents.

When President Nixon went to China in 1971, and James Reston of the New York Times wrote about his experiences after an appendectomy using acupuncture for pain relief, I saw another procedure which I could use in my practice of anesthesiology. I immediately started to learn about the subject of acupuncture, and through the encouragement of my friend, Frank Z. Warren, M.D. began to involve myself in the use of acupuncture therapy for the relief of pain. I was able to follow my patients, both in hypnotherapy and acupuncture, by survey for a period of three years, and I am convinced that both hypnotherapy and acupuncture are of value in treating the patient with pain.

I retired from the practice of anesthesiology in 1984, and taught Statistics and Research Methods in the graduate program of Health Sciences at The Wichita State University. I was not involved in either hypnotherapy or acupuncture therapy for the next four years. When I was retired from the University, a program was started at The Olive W. Garvey Center in Wichita for those patients who had chronic illnesses over a long period of time, and who were not getting relief by conventional methods of therapy. We have incorporated a pain track in our practice, and I have begun to use hypnotherapy and acupuncture as a part of the treatment for our patients. The need for review made me think of a method in which I could train myself both in techniques for hypnotherapy as well as acupuncture.

The notes and diagrams used to retrain myself in hypnosis and acupuncture were put together, and the idea of writing a book came to mind. The techniques and semantics are those that I use in my practice, and I hope that it will prove of value to those who read the book. There are many techniques and procedures that can be used, but this book is written especially for the patient with pain. The majority of patients are those with complaints of pain, particularly chronic pain, who have gone through many physicians, medications, and suggestions, and I hope that their introduction to hypnosis and acupuncture will be the end of their search for relief.

I would like to thank Hugh D. Riordan, M.D. for his interest in my pursuit of therapy using hypnosis and acupuncture, and encouraging me to write this book. I would also like to thank Barbara Nichols for her help in transposing the material I had on my computer to the final form, and Lisa Hostetler for her assistance in drawing the illustrations for this book. I hope that there is as much pleasure in reading the book as I had in writing it.

M. M. Tinterow, M.D., Ph.D.

INTRODUCTION

This book will not be a technical treatise on the subject of pain. Much has been written on the subject, both in medical journals and in magazines that adorn the checkout counters of the supermarkets. However, the material and information which you will find in the following pages of this book are written for the nonprofessional in everyday language. You won't need a medical dictionary to learn the definition of medical terms, and the approach will not be to give you the various treatments for the relief of pain. This book has been my association with the relief of pain over the past 45 years in the practice of medicine and the specialty of Anesthesiology.

Every book that one reads tries to establish for the reader the fact that there are certain treatments for certain types of pain. If that is the case, we have found many definitive treatments for the relief of pain, some orthodox and others unorthodox. What one has to understand primarily is that the sensation of pain is subjective, and as a consequence of this, the myriad of therapies prescribed fits each and everyone of the subjective complaints of the patient.

I am a retired anesthesiologist, and anesthesiology has always been a specialty in the practice of medicine that deals with the relief of pain. As the study of medicine grew in both technical skills and knowledge of the human body, many additional modalities presented themselves as aids in the relief of pain. Hypnotherapy, biofeedback, acupuncture, trigger point injections of local anesthetic agents, Tens units, TM, Yoga, and many others became popular as information about their success filtered down to the general public through the Reader's Digest, Redbook, National Enquirer, and the Star magazine. The glowing accounts of success of these measures assured widespread use in the relief of pain.

What actually is pain? Why are there so many gradations of pain? How can we really measure pain? Can we describe organic pain, and at the same time describe psychogenic pain in the same terms? When we watch television each day, at the commercial break, we are liable to see the comparison of the various analgetics taken to relieve headaches. Each performer on the commercial, with a smile on his/her face describes the severe pain caused by the headache, and how the product advertised is so much better than any other because of this or that medication that is present in larger amounts. Did you know that there are medications that work only from 6 A.M. to 6 P.M., and after 6 P.M. you have to take that medication to which has been added a P.M. factor to help from 6 P.M. to 6 A.M?

What if I were to make the following statement, "There is no such thing as pain"? I am afraid that I would have to run for my life, because of the many people who would take exception to that statement. There are many definitions of pain. My definition of pain is the "projection of a symptom complex to accomplish a means to an end." Would you accept that definition? Think for a moment and try to recall your last headache? When did it occur? Did it follow any specific pattern? Did it occur at a particular time of a certain day? Have you kept track of specific incidents that occurred at that time, and have you recorded those incidents that happened at that time to see if they coincided with incidents that happened at an earlier time? Do these incidents relate to the onset of a headache? Do you wake up with a headache after sleeping a full and restful night?

Why do some people have a slight headache and others one that is rather severe? Why are some headaches described as being a sick headache, and others as making you feel as though your eyeballs are being pushed out of their sockets? Why do some people only complain of headaches starting Friday night, and others complain starting Monday morning? I have seen patients who have complained of continuous headaches for the last ten years, and have been seeking relief for that period of time. Why do headaches begin in the occipital region of the skull and then travel in all directions over the entire skull? Why do headaches feel as though there was a tight band around your forehead squeezing tighter and tighter as the headaches get more severe? Why are headaches only on one side, either in the temporal area or the frontal area? Why are some headaches behind the eyes, and others on the top of the head pressing down into the skull?

Let us try a little experiment that will explain to you the interpretation of pain in your body. Sit down comfortably in a chair and close your eyes. I will then take a pen and on the back of your hand I will mark an "X." I will now take a pin, and I will stick you in the middle of the "X." With your eyes closed, you will be able to identify the sensation caused by the sticking of the pin. The response will be,"Ouch, you're sticking me." Then, I will raise the skin on the back of your hand at the mark,"X," between two fingers and pinch you. You will respond by saying, "Ouch, you're pinching me." If you place a cube of ice over the "X," you will say that it is cold, and if you are touched with a hot object, you will describe the response that you are being burned. An incision with a sharp object elicits, "Ouch , you're cutting me." How does one minute area allow you to interpret all those sensations? What is located there to differentiate the differences to painful stimuli?

There are nerve endings under the skin where the mark was placed and each stimulus elicits a response by creating an electrical current that travels from the nerve ending of a smaller nerve to the next larger nerve, then to the spinal cord. In the spinal cord are spinothalamic tracts that ascend up into the conscious area of the brain located on the right side. There, the electrical impulse is interpreted by experiential learning. You had in the past perceived that sensation, and you stored it away in your subconscious center to recall it when it was needed. There is nothing mysterious about it, since all pain is learned. You have to complain about the pain for anyone to know that you are having pain. Nothing on the top of your head lights up to give a sign. It is a subjective response. Distract your attention, and the pain is gone. Recall it, and the pain returns. We could discuss this point for many pages without reaching any conclusion; however, the reports of many operative conditions being performed with only hypnosis as the anesthesia being used seems to bear out the point about what pain actually is, and what we are going to do to eliminate it.

Neural pathways are always traced when pain is explained, but to the individual who has pain, this is not an answer. Collins, in his textbook, PRINCIPLES OF ANESTHESIOLOGY states, "In the evaluation of any pain-relieving measure, the nature of the pain must be considered. A complaint of pain which brings the patient to a physician is a personal sensory experience, unique for that specific individual. As a subjective experience, it is at best difficult to evaluate, and there is naturally wide variation in the interpretation and reaction to the pain." To the individual, the pain is real. It is excruciating, and relief is being sought from the physician.

There is a need for the individual to have pain. Not only do we see that there can be a response by the subject to the initial stimulus, but the reaction of the individual is dependent on the interpretation of that sensation. What is happening at the time of the stimulus will determine the severity of the sensation. Everyone will agree that there are times when we can distract our attention from the situation, and as a result, the perception of pain is diminished. Likewise, through the use of suggestions, we can ease the interpretation of the stimulus. How many times have we, as parents, had our children fall and sustain an injury which made them cry? What were the words which soothed them at that time? The words that we used were: "Come over here and let me kiss it and make it well." The crying would stop, and the child would return to his/her play without another sound.

Suggestion is very important in symptom control; however, this does not mean that its use can be a panacea for the control of the discomfort from which you suffer. Too many charlatans have made the use of suggestions available, and it is easy to see how this approach can attract so many individuals. The patient, who has visited the physician on numerous occasions to seek relief from what is perceived as severe pain will try anything in order to obtain relief. It doesn't matter whether it is practical or not. The hope that relief is in sight will have an effect on the patient. What can a patient do if all that he/she is told is that there is nothing that can be found to explain the pain? "It must be in your mind." The pain is psychogenic in origin, and since no one wants to accept this fact, the patient will immediately seek another source for relief of that pain.

From the very beginning of my work with hypnosis, I have been interested in the history of the subject. I am of the opinion that knowing the history, and understanding the development of the methods and techniques used, allows for an indepth understanding of what training is taking place at that time. This led me to becoming a collector of books on the subject of Mesmerism, Animal Magnetism and Hypnosis. My collection of 640 rare books on the subject was donated to the Rare Books Collection at The Wichita State University in 1982. Interested individuals may use these references if they are interested in the history of Hypnosis.

My interest in pain relief evolved from my career as an anesthesiologist. There is little personal involvement with the surgical patient other than a preoperative visit. Around the late 1950s there was a renewed resurgence in the subject of hypnotism. Courses were offered throughout the country, and I enrolled to learn the subject. At that time I was only interested in the use of hypnosis as a substitute for the anesthetic agents that were used at that time. That same year, I used hypnoanesthesia for an open heart operation on a 15 year-old girl which lasted for four and one-half hours. Using hypnosis alone, or in conjunction with narcotic analgetics, other procedures such as Cesarean section, vaginal hysterectomy, abdominal oophorectomy, vein ligation, change of burn dressings, a second open heart operation, breast biopsy, and many others were done. These patients were chosen because of allergic manifestations to anesthetic agents, or anatomical abnormalities which would interfere with respiration or circulation of the patients. In 1970, C.C. Thomas, Publishers, Springfield, Illinois, published FOUNDATIONS OF

HYPNOSIS: From Mesmer to Freud, a historical development of hypnosis using selections from many of the early books in my collection. I am of the opinion that Mesmer and other early nineteenth century physicians have something to teach the physician of today. Today, the physicians, who practice Holistic medicine are rediscovering the importance of body, mind and spirit that the Mesmerists of earlier centuries took for granted.

Try to relax as you read this book. Chances are that your eyes will get heavy, and you will fall asleep. It is not the hypnotic spell that is being cast, instead it is the intense concentration that will probably result in the tiring of the eyes, and slowly your eyes will close, and you will be in a state of hypnosis. DON'T BELIEVE IT. It won't happen, but that is a good way to start, and if you will turn the page, you will be told the myths and false beliefs that we have against the subject of HYPNOSIS.

1

"Look into my eyes! Your eyes are growing heavy. You are getting sleepy." This statement has been used over and over again as an introduction to starting a session in hypnosis. Nothing is going to happen. Nothing can happen. You are in control of your own actions, and no one can make you close your eyes. Today the word, hypnosis, still has the connotation of mystery and black magic. The word hypnosis is derived from the Greek word, "HYPNOS," meaning a state of sleep. However, there is no connection between hypnosis and sleep. The only resemblance is that the subject is sitting with eyes closed, but there are also states of hypnosis in which the subject may have their eyes open throughout the entire session. What do you feel like in a state of hypnosis? Is there a different feeling? Forget all of your preconceived ideas about what you think it really is, and try to learn the facts about what it is, how it acts, and how it can be used to good advantage.

Remember this fact. No one is going to hypnotize you. I have never hypnotized anyone with the exception of myself. All hypnosis is self hypnosis. I repeat—all hypnosis is self hypnosis. All that one can do is to show the subject how the state of hypnosis can be entered into by themselves. Today, there is real doubt if the words "hypnotic trance" indicate a true state or just a frame of mind reacting to suggestion. Hypnosis is a state of hypersuggestibility. If you examine hypnosis clinically, you find that it doesn't look, act or feel the way you think it should. The question that you have to ask yourself is, "What do I want to do with hypnosis?" Remember, no one can hypnotize anyone, and so the feeling of power that you want to place within yourself won't be realized if you try to practice hypnosis by yourself. You will never be able to give a suggestion to a subject unless they are willing to accept the suggestion. At all times and in all degrees of hypnosis, the subject has full and complete power of selectivity, and reacts only to those suggestions which are responsible and pleasing to them.

Then why do we see people who are in a presumed state of hypnosis do crazy things, like crawling around on their hands and feet and barking like a dog, or eating an onion while thinking it is an apple. Those individuals are only reacting to the suggestions that have been given to them by the hypnotist. These suggestions are pleasing to the individual or else the individual would have refused the suggestions. The individual who volunteers to be a subject usually has an outgoing personality, is an extrovert, and enjoys being the center of attention. Those who are just the opposite, an introvert, wouldn't have volunteered in the first place. Remember—in all cases—the subject retains selectivity.

In the final analysis, even though the subject is amenable to suggestion, it is the subject who is in complete control. Let a crisis arise, and the element of self preservation comes into play. The subject will then reject the suggestion and continue in the state or will reject the suggestion by coming out of the hypnotic state. There are four criteria that are necessary for an individual to enter into a state of relaxation through suggestion: (1) the desire or willingness to be hypnotized, (2) the ability to concentrate, (3) average intelligence, and (4) freedom from fear.

The person in a trance state has complete possession of his faculties—he can hear, think for himself, speak, feel, see, and although he may look unconscious, he is completely aware and can cooperate at all times. He has the ability to give himself selective awareness or unawareness at will. Most people think that you enter into a state of unconsciousness when you are hypnotized. This is not the case. You are unconscious to your surroundings. It is as though you are watching a movie on television, become so engrossed in the movie, that the phone may ring but you do not hear it. Only when it interrupts your thoughts, do you then go to answer the phone. When you see people react to a suggestion, then you realize that every individual reacts in a different way. You should be able to respond to those suggestions and know what to do. Everyone should not attempt to use suggestions on others. Do you know what to do after an individual has entered into a state of hypnosis? There is no doubt in my mind that induction techniques can be learned by anyone, but now that the subject is in a state of suggestibility, what are you going to do next? Are you going to try to remove symptoms that the subject needs to combat anxiety and frustration? This is better left to the professional. In the later chapters,

I will give you several induction techniques that you can use for your own self hypnosis. Use it only on yourself for relaxation, and the ability to meet the challenges of everyday life.

No one can thoroughly learn hypnosis by observing it on others. You must experience it yourself to know how different it is from the things that you have read or heard. You will find hypnosis a pleasant state, and you will probably want to try it. Instead of resisting, as your knowledge about the subject increases and your fear decreases, and the fallacies about hypnosis are cleared up, you will reach the state where you will want to try it for yourself. Most everyone can be hypnotized if they have the desire and have average intelligence. There are about three percent of the population who are imbeciles and morons, and consequently, if you want to brag about being an individual who can't be hypnotized, you know in what percentage of the population you place yourself. Self-preservation governs the subject who is in a state of relaxation, and that is why no one has been injured in a state of hypnosis. Hypnosis has been in the hands of charlatans, quacks, amateurs, and fakes for a long period of time, but you still have to find the first case on record which will bear investigation where a person has done harm in a suggestible state.

There is little doubt that a person can be talked into committing a crime without hypnosis as easily as he could with hypnosis. It simply would be the long way around, hypnosis could not be blamed for the crime. If you don't have the desire to be hypnotized you won't be. The consent of the subject is necessary and in addition, the subject has to be able to communicate and understand what is going on at the time of the session. But above all, the most important criteria for entering into a state of suggestibility is freedom from fear; fear that you may not come out of the state, and fear that you will be made to do unpleasurable acts. You will not do anything that is immoral, illegal, or unethical. Again, remember that you are in control of your own mind. The thing to bear in mind is that hypnosis is a state of highly perfected and increased awareness. Everything we do in the hypnotic situation is a vastly magnified bit of what we ordinarily do with many times greater impact than what occurs in ordinary life. The problem is that after we hypnotize an individual, most of the untrained do not then know what to do.

What happens when one attempts to induce a particular reaction in a human being? If the hypnotist is producing under certain circumstances conditioned responses and conditioning, he must be aware that this is happening, and be familiar with the consequences of conditioning and what some of the by-products of conditioned behavior are. An essential element in the field of hypnosis that is needed today is more concentrated and intensive research on the basic aspects of hypnosis. It becomes the responsibility of those who are going to use hypnosis also to be responsible for observing what they do, and attempting to report and (within the limits of their competence) to undertake those types of research studies which will lead to greater understanding about what is being done.

It is really unfortunate that those who are doing hypnosis fail to appreciate the full meaning of what they are doing. That is why periods occur in which enthusiasm for hypnosis and for the utilization of hypnotic techniques in medical treatment and in psychotherapy reach great heights and then decline. Freud abandoned hypnosis after a few years, although he gained many of the insights which led him to the practice of psychoanalysis, because within it he saw the unraveling of the human mind. Today, hypnosis is no longer concerned with the mind alone but with the totality of human experience.

Under hypnosis, an individual enters into a relationship with another individual, the hypnotist. This is not something that is done easily, and it is not something which is done without resistance. Resistance in hypnosis always exists, although it may not always be recognized. An awareness of resistance is always the first step in understanding the nature of the hypnotic relationship and may reveal important clues as to how this relationship which has been established can best be used. Actually, responses due to hypnotic intervention are not necessarily limited to the words or the direct suggestions that are employed by the hypnotist, but may be intermediate responses determined by the reaction of the individual subject to the meaning of the hypnotic communication.

Not every medical practitioner is suitable to becoming a hypnotist. During the 1950s and 1960s, every physician thought that he would use hypnosis in his practice. Many three-day weekend classes were held by physicians and lay hypnotists who travelled around the country visiting city after city introducing the art of hypnotism to the local physicians, dentists, and psychologists. It is true that the personal magnetic fluid, which used to be considered necessary, is a superfluous myth, but everyone does not possess the characteristics and capabilities of enthusiasm, consistency, and the ability to invent original ideas. By far, the most potent factor which stands in the way of success is the want of personal interest and of personal initiative. One must be wholeheartedly involved in using hypnosis, and not attempt to use hypnosis in an automatic sort of way, following out a preconceived scheme. The individual hypnotist will rapidly have poor results to record as soon as the fascination of the novelty of the thing has passed. The hypnotist will go to sleep himself more and more, and his patients will be influenced less and less.

A second factor which prevents success is mistrust, nervousness, fear that others will laugh at him, fear that the hypnotized person will simulate misgivings and doubts of all kinds. This second factor, which at first is the most formidable, disappears as soon as one gains experience, and then the first factor makes itself felt to the full extent, and must continuously be combatted. One can frequently notice, when one is depressed or tired, that one achieves fewer results, for this weakness of the hypnotist is unconsciously recognized by the brain of the individual who is being hypnotized.

One should approach the person to be hypnotized quite naturally with intent on one purpose, and that is to hypnotize the individual. It should be explained to the subject that there is nothing unnatural or uncanny about the state of hypnosis, and that it is a characteristic of the nervous system which applies to everyone. He will neither be influenced or under the power of the hypnotist, and he will not fall asleep. The hypnotist should avoid long speeches or explanations, and the subject should be allowed to relax for a few moments with total silence around him so that he may acclimate himself to the surroundings. One should try to secure the trust and inclination of the person to be hypnotized.

At the beginning the hypnotist should avoid a commanding tone of voice, and should be able to use deflections in his voice to suit the occasion. The phenomena of suggestion should be represented, especially to the educated persons, as arising quite naturally out of themselves. The person who is being hypnotized should not be mentally stimulated or excited, and a condition of expected tension should be avoided. Some individuals are afraid that they can't be hypnotized and give themselves autosuggestion, which is frequently difficult to overcome. Many of the subjects do not achieve deep relaxation at the first attempt, but an explanation of the conditioning effect of hypnotherapy should allay all fears that the hypnosis is not working.

The hypnotist must not do any harm by suggestion, which can occur during the first session of hypnotherapy. Persons who are anxious and nervous are apt to imagine autosuggestion of harmful actions as a result of the first hypnotherapy session. This is particularly likely if they have learned a lot of this kind of thing from newspapers or other people. They become giddy after the hypnosis, or they feel themselves dazed, or they have a feeling of fear or even have a headache. One must interfere in this type of reaction, and explain to the subject that these conditions are a result of anxiety and concern over the condition that is being treated. Ignoring this can result in unintentional damages caused by hypnotherapy. One must always suggest perfect health, cheerful mood, sleep, good appetite, and the strengthening of the will. Suggestions towards increasing motivation and elevation of self-esteem are helpful in ending the session.

If suggestion fails after four or five sessions, the hypnotist should not continue with the subject. It sometimes succeeds later, or if another hypnotist tries. The hypnotist should try to achieve maximum benefit in a few sessions. The hypnotist must reduce the number of sessions gradually, and then give the subject a rest from the sessions. If there are no results with the sessions, the hypnotist and the hypnotized become tired. Do not hesitate to use other therapeutic means with the hypnosis, and then gradually wean the subject from the alternative type of therapy.

2

A study of the history of hypnosis is necessary in order to have a clear knowledge of what it is or is not. In the long course of its history, hypnotism has been the frequent trade of the unscientific investigator, and, indeed, all of the charlatans and quacks at one time or another have endeavored to make some use of it. Its peculiar attraction for these men lay in the fact that the ordinary run of mankind knew nothing of the hypnotic state. In the narrowness of their philosophy, they were willing to attribute to the supernatural or to the unknown, all that they, in their ignorance, could not appreciate or understand.

The history of hypnotism begins almost at the beginning of civilization. In the book of Genesis we read the statement, "And the Lord caused a deep sleep to fall upon Adam and removed a rib from him." Could this have been "hypnoanesthesia"? There were techniques that were used by the Egyptians, the Greeks, and the Romans which present a striking similarity to the techniques adopted by modern hypnotists. In Egyptian lore, there are stories of the goddess Isis standing with her hands uplifted and evidently about to "pass" over her subjects. The EBERS PAPYRUS, which gives us some account of the medical methods practiced in Egypt before 1552 B.C., mentions the laying on of hands on the head of the patient as a part of the treatment.

Asclepiades was in the habit of putting frenzied persons to sleep by rubbing, and when these frictions were prolonged, the patient was plunged into a deep lethargy. Tacitus and Suetonis testified to the cures performed by the Emperor Vespasian. Finally, St. Augustine told of a priest he knew, who could reduce himself to a state not to be distinguished from death. Everyone has heard of the cures due to "royal touch." Numerous cures were affected in this manner by the early kings of France, and the touch was still in vogue in Queen Anne's time. It seems to have been first exercised by the Scandinavian princes and princesses, and particularly by St. Olaf, who was supposed to have reigned from 1020 to 1035.

In the middle ages, priests were seen exorcising the devil. This is the beginning of a new form of suggestive therapeutics. Everyone who lived in the 15th and 16th centuries believed in witchcraft. Paracelsus introduced a "weapon salve" which could be rubbed on a weapon after a wound had been inflicted, and by virtue of its great powers, it would ease the wound. There were other strange and unusual stories of individuals who had concocted cures that had a relationship to the imagery which was portrayed during a so-called curative session.

Many of the phenomena that were demonstrated are connected with the oracles, or with the most learned physicians. Because of the source, people either did not look for any explanation or attributed the result to a supernatural power. The first traces of any system for these phenomena appeared at the end of the Middle Ages, and this system grew out of the doctrines of astrology. Many of the famous men of that time were at work on the subject. Prominent among the writers were Paracelsus, Athanasius Kircher, van Helmont, Sebastian Wirdig, and many others.

All of these men attempted, in various ways, to demonstrate the existence of a universal magnetic force by which the reciprocal action of bodies upon each other, and particularly the phenomenon of the human body and mind, were to be explained. One individual was capable of producing an effect upon the mind and organs of other individuals. Pomponatius, Professor of Philosophy at Padua, was born in Mantua in 1462 and died in 1525. He sought to prove that sickness and disease were curable by means of "magnetism" existing in each person. He calculated that the force upon the imagination and the will within a person could affect the blood and the spirits which, in turn, would produce results as the disease was cast out of the body.

John Baptist von Helmont was born in Brussels in the year 1577. He was educated in the medical profession but spent his life in chemical research. The discovery of laudanum, or the spirit of hartshorn, and their volatile salts are due to his research. He also discovered the existence of the aeriform fluids, to which he gave the name "gas," a name which is still retained. He defined magnetism as an occult power which bodies exert over each other at a distance, whether by attraction or repulsion. In the middle of the eighteenth century, many men were attracted to the whole question of magnetism by witnessing the wonderful "cures" performed by Father Hehl, a Jesuit. The cures were supposed to be due to the subtle influence on body fluid by magnetism, which was imparted to patients from steel plates and magnets prepared especially for that purpose.

Franz Anton Mesmer came upon the scene with his theories on Animal Magnetism, and published his first dissertation in 1766. The work of Mesmer and his disciples was the beginning of the development of hypnosis, and is the first chapter of the history of hypnosis.

Mesmer was born at Weiler-on-the-Rhine in the year 1734. He studied medicine in his youth and settled as a physician in Vienna, where he ultimately married advantageously. In 1766 he wrote a dissertation when he received his degree, "De Planetarium Influxu," in which he stated that he believed health is based on a fluidum, that this fluid comes from magnets, and from the astral bodies. He studied further, and engaged in arguments with Father Gassner who believed in exorcising the devil. Mesmer tried to convince his colleagues that what he was doing was related to magnetism, and every scientist should know about magnetism. At this time new concepts about magnetic phenomena and electricity were being discussed. His dissertation drew much ridicule and professional opposition. The attempt to account for this influence led him to make the experiments which introduced him to the facts with which his name has been associated. At first he worked entirely with magnets and obtained some cures by this means, but he was much persecuted for his audacity. He established a private hospital for the relief of destitute individuals. He soon came to the conclusion that the magnetic rods with which the first experiments were made, served only as conductors for the fluid emanating from his own body. To this he at once gave the name Animal Magnetism, and theorized boldly concerning its diffusion through nature. But he was accused of deceiving the public, and of having magnetic rods concealed about his person—an accusation which was very amusing, in view of the fact that, when he really used magnetic rods, he was ridiculed for expecting to obtain curative results by such means. His reputation was assailed and his fortune impaired. He moved from Vienna to Paris in 1777 to seek a more favorable theater for the development of his experiments. The theory put forward rested on Mesmer's conviction that there was a reciprocal influence between the heavenly bodies, the earth and animated beings. The medium of this influence he perceived to be a subtle fluid pervading the whole universe, which from its nature is capable of receiving, propagating and communicating every impulse of motion. Mesmer's suggestions to this effect were treated by men of science in Paris with contempt.

The public meanwhile became interested, to some extent, in new ideas, as the fame of the various cures had been spread around. Various persons testified that Mesmer had cured them, but the public journals ridiculed him, and the medical profession reviled him. In 1781 he published a work entitled "Precis Historique des Faits relatif au Magnetisme Animal." The opposition he encountered only stimulated his own enthusiasm, and led him to proclaim magnetism as a panacea.

Mesmer felt so strongly about the magnetism that he declared that there is but one health, one disease, one remedy. He established a secret society, under the name of "The Harmony," where he initiated pupils into the mystery of his process, taking from them fees of hundreds of louis d'or each. He took fees from wealthy people and is said to have remitted them when would-be pupils were less prosperous.

In 1779, Mesmer published a dissertation, "Memoire sur la decourvete du Magnetisme Animal" (Discovery of Animal Magnetism) in which he promised to make a system on the subject which would revolutionize not only the thinking in medicine but in philosophy. Struck with the clearness and accuracy of his reasonings, the extraordinary and unquestionable cures he performed, some of the greatest and most prominent physicians and philosophers of France became his converts.

As Mesmer became more popular, he became much more sought after by the rich. To be mesmerized was considered to be quite a social thing at the time. Mesmer developed what he called a "baquet." He was so busy that he couldn't see all of his patients so he placed some holes in a barrel and then filled the barrel with iron filings and rods were placed through the holes to the outside. The iron bars were supposed to be magnetized since Mesmer had touched each one of them. Techniques differ, but anything works when the patient believes it will have an effect. These were magnetized bars, and when Mesmer would point a wand at the patient holding on to the rod, the patient would develop a mesmeric crisis. This was acute hysterical excitement. Mesmer believed that, only when the patient was in a crisis, a curative effect and healing occurred. The patient was convinced that something was flowing into them, and so was the practitioner, and this type of interpersonal relationship produced the Mesmeric "crisis."

In 1784 a Royal Commission was appointed by King Louis XVI to inquire into the claims advanced in behalf of animal magnetism. This report was unfavorable, although the general body of the commissioners acknowledged the effects produced by the magnetic treatment, but repudiated Mesmer's theory of a fluid and preferred hypothesis concerning the actions of the magnetic application. Mesmer eventually retired to Switzerland in disgust, and died at an advanced age in 1815, closing his career as it had begun, by practicing magnetic cures gratuitously for the benefit of the poor.

Among the earliest of Mesmer's disciples, the Marquis Chastenet de Puysegur wrote extensively on the subject of his own prolonged and varied practice as a curative magnetist. The whole collection of writings embodies an immense accumulation of experiences of persons clairvoyant during illness. He gives examples of his cases, but it seems strange that he never apparently investigated the extent to which the clairvoyant perceptions he evoked could be directed towards other subjects besides those having to do with physical illness. In the beginning mesmerism was introduced to the whole world in reference almost exclusively to its medical aspect, and it was reserved for later investigators to bring its psychological importance into view.

Dr. James Esdaile's "Mesmerism in India" is a record of extraordinary success in the application of mesmerism to his surgical practice at the government hospital in Calcutta. The book was published in 1842. It includes not only minute surgical reports of operations performed upon mesmerized patients without any suffering or consciousness of what was taking place on their part, but also collaborative testimony from many of the most distinguished people in Calcutta at that time, who were called in by Dr. Esdaile to be present and witness the surgical procedures.

In a brief account of Mesmer's life in the eighth edition of the Encyclopaedia Brittanica he is represented as a detected impostor, and without one word to indicate that there is even any considerable body of opinion opposed to that view. It refers to the fact that the disciples of animal magnetism attempted to check the advance of their enemies by forming themselves into societies. Mesmer, more polite, escaped amid the general confusion, carrying with him a subscription of 340,000 francs, and at the same time a secret for which that sum had been given to him. For the moment the mesmeric fluid theory is altogether out of fashion, and the most recent inquirers have set out to work and try to rediscover the facts that were written in the last century. It is time for those who want to investigate the validity and reliability of mesmerism to try and observe the facts that will lay a foundation for understanding the various aspects of this science.

James Braid (1795-1860) was an English surgeon who inaugurated modern hypnotism, the word itself being introduced by him. His theories were adopted by Broca, Charcot, Liebault, and Bernheim. NEURYPNOLOGY, or the Rationale of Nervous Sleep, was the first book actually published with hypnosis as the subject. Braid carried on the work of Mesmer in England, although he recognized that the art of magnetism was actually the result of suggestion and was not what was previously believed. Braid's work is monumental as a contribution to modern hypnotism. Modern theories still trace their beginning to the work which Braid accomplished with his practice of hypnosis.

Jean Martin Charcot, who was the greatest of the French neurologists insisted that hypnosis was a neurosis, a form of nerve pathology. Charcot would again introduce hypnosis into the halls of medicine and make it respectable. Later, Sigmund Freud became involved with Charcot's explanation of hypnosis, and in it he was very impressed with the fact that when a patient was hypnotized, the patient was not aware of what was going on. Freud began to postulate that something was going on in the subconscious. This became a lead to modern psychoanalysis.

The popularity of hypnosis seemed to drop to a low level after Freud started using psychoanalysis. The present era of hypnosis begins with such investigators as Hull and Williams. Others who have pursued an interest in both the experimental and clinical approaches to hypnosis are Wells, Erickson, LeCron, Kline, Weitzenhoffer, Rosen, Raginsky and Wolberg, as well as others too numerous to mention. They have developed many sophisticated techniques that have advanced the knowledge of hypnosis. However, simple techniques which I will describe can offer as much as can the more sophisticated techniques. Books describing these many varied approaches to hypnosis can be found in books that have been published to date.

3

Most subjects have a fear of the word "hypnosis." It is very important that we allay those fears in the individual. We must reduce anxiety in the subject, and when you explain what you are planning to do, tell it in a language which he understands. If the subject brings up the word, hypnosis, don't try to avoid answering the question. The anxiety which is created may prove to be a block to the successful use of hypnotherapy. The hypnotist must have confidence in knowing that he can induce a trance state in the subject. Most of the time there is an interaction between the hypnotist and the subject. There is a "rapport" established from the beginning; the same kind of reactions to the hypnotist which they have learned toward authoritative figures in childhood are manifested toward the hypnotist. The hypnotist does become the parent figure, and he does hypnotize by assuming that role.

When is success realized in hypnosis? The stage hypnotist seems to be successful in hypnotizing his subjects. How does he work? How does he know that he will find a successful subject so that he can complete his act? A brief explanation will suffice. The audience with which the hypnotist is dealing is usually one in which there are those individuals who are extrovert in nature. If they were not, when the hypnotist asks for volunteers from the audience, an individual who is introverted would not volunteer. The hypnotist usually asks for volunteers, the number of which can be divided by three. He then will begin with a test for suggestibility, asking the volunteers to put their feet on the floor, palms down in their lap, and sit comfortably in the chair.

He then asks the subjects to close their eyes and put their arms in front of them. Then he asks them to imagine that he is placing a weight on their right arm below the elbow. Then he asks them to imagine that he is placing a weight on the left arm below the elbow. He then suggests that he is placing increasing amounts of weight for their arms to support, and finally suggests that the weight is so heavy that their arms are beginning to drop. He looks for those whose arms begin to slowly drop, and this is usually a sign of hypnotic suggestibility. From the group, he usually will have three or four who will be suggestibile, and with whom he will continue to work to make his show successful. He emphasizes relaxation, and suggests that the subjects are getting sleepy. He continues to watch for those who constantly move in their chairs, and who do not respond to the further suggestions. These subjects are then excused, and he continues with his act.

There are many approches he can use in hypnotizing the individuals. The simple technique of eye fixation usually produces a hypnotic state easier than does other techniques. Usually the hypnotist ends up with one or two excellent subjects, and then continues suggesting that the individual will get down on his hands and knees and bark like a dog, responding to other suggestions that mimic the action of a dog. Even though the individual is conscious, he will obey the hypnotist. The stage hypnotist is a very good inducer of trance states. He does so primarily through fear. Fear can cause rapid entering into a trance state, but it is not that successful in maintaining a hypnotic state. Let us proceed with induction through the use of the eye fixation method, learning the semantics which are used in induction techniques. After that, you will learn how it feels to be in a relaxed state.

"Sit comfortable in your chair..." (If there is a recliner present it may be tilted to the first position)

"Take in a real deep breath and blow it out slowly..."

"Feel yourself relaxing from the top of your head to the tips of your toes..."

"Find a spot on the opposite wall, or on the ceiling above, and fix your eyes on that spot..."

"Now, take in another breath, releasing all anxieties and tensions..."

"Now I want you to notice in your own mind and physically as well..."

"that your feet are getting heavy, and heavier and heavier..."

"So heavy, that you can't lift them off the floor..."

"Heavier and heavier, heavier and heavier..."

"So heavy, that they are not a part of you..."

"But they get heavier than that, and heavier and heavier..."

"and suddenly they relax and grow real light..."

"And then your legs and your knees..."

"grow heavy, and heavier and heavier..."

"And heavier and heavier, that you can't lift them off of the floor..."

"and heavier and heavier..."

"that they feel like two rods of iron, they are so heavy..."

"But they get even heavier than that..."

"and suddenly, they, too, relax and grow real light..."

"and then your thighs and your hips and your abdomen grows real heavy..."

"and heavier and heavier..."

"so heavy that you feel like you can't lift your body out of the chair..."

"But your body gets even heavier than that..."

"and so heavy, so very heavy, so very heavy..."

"and heavier, and heavier..."

"and suddenly from your waist down to the tips of your toes..."

"your whole body relaxes and grows real light..."

"And now your arms, your shoulders and your chest grow real heavy..."

"and heavier, and heavier..."

"and so heavy, so very heavy..."

"and your breathing gets deeper, and deeper..."

"deeper and deeper, deeper and deeper..."

"and your whole body feels real heavy..."

"heavier and heavier..."

"and suddenly your whole body from your neck down to the tips of your toes relaxes and grows real light..."

"And then your neck and your face grow real heavy..."

"And your eyes are growing real heavy..."

"and your eyes are getting drowsy..."

"and heavier and heavier..."

"that they are starting to close..."

"slowly closing, slowly closing, slowly closing..

"All the way down, all the way down, all the w. down..."

"So let your eyes stay closed, your eyes are closed...

"And then let yourself, both physically and mentally..."

"feel as though you are going into a deep state of sleep..."

(Clap both hands)...

"Deep asleep, deep, deep, asleep, deep asleep, deep asleep, deep asleep..."

"Completely asleep, completely asleep, completely asleep..."

"From the top of your head, to the tips of your toes, completely relaxed, completely relaxed..."

"So completely relaxed from the top of your head to the tips of your toes, that nothing will bother you, and nothing will harm you..."

"Completely relaxed, completely relaxed..."

"Deep asleep, deep asleep, deep asleep..."

"Completely relaxed, completely relaxed, completely relaxed..."

"Deep, deep, deep asleep..."

"Completely relaxed, completely relaxed, completely relaxed..."

"From the top of your head to the tips of your toes, and not a single muscle will move, and your body will feel as though it is floating on a cloud..."

"completely relaxed, completely relaxed, completely relaxed..."

"And now, in a moment when I tell you to and not before, I want you to take in a deep breath..."

"blow it all the way out..."

"Keep your eyes closed..."

"and picture yourself stepping onto an escalator that is going all the way down into a basement..."

"going down and down and down, into the greatest depth of relaxation that you have ever imagined..."

"down, and down, and down..."

"getting more relaxed and more relaxed as you go down, down, down..."

"So now, let's take in a deep breath, blow it all the way out, keep your eyes closed, and let's go....... DOWN..."

(Clap your hands)

"Down, down, down, down, deeper, and deeper, and down..."

"Down, down, down...deeper and deeper and down, down, down..."

"Completely relaxed, completely relaxed, and down, down, and down..."

"From the top of your head to the tips of your toes, not a single muscle will move, and your body will feel as though it is floating on a cloud..."

"Down, down, down..."

"Down, down, down...completely relaxed, completely relaxed..."

"down, down, down, completely relaxed..."

"And now, in a moment when I tell you, and not before..."

"I want you to take in a real deep breath, blow it all the way out, keep your eyes closed..."

"and when I count to three and clap my hands..."

"I want you to remove from your subconscious mind, all the tensions and anxieties that you have built up concerning the problems that you are facing today..."

"So now...take in a deep breath, blow it all the way out, keep your eyes closed, and one...two... and three...(clap your hands)..."

"I want you to remove from your subconscious mind all tensions and anxieties regarding the problems that you are having with (whatever the problem, symptom, or illness might be)..."

"and I want you to use all the suggestions that you will be given concerning the removal of such symptoms and problems..."

"I want you to be completely relaxed both physically and mentally, and feel a surge of energy and agressiveness enter into your body..."

"Your body will feel so good..."

"there will be a warmth surging throughout your body..."

"Inside and outside, you will feel completely relaxed both physically and mentally..."

"So now, let's take in a deep breath, keep your eyes closed, and one...two...and three..."

(Clap your hands)

"Completely relaxed..."

"Completely relaxed..."

"Completely relaxed..."

"Now I want you to remove from your subconscious mind all tensions and anxieties that you have built up..."

"And I want you to use the suggestions that I give you to benefit you in whatever way that you see fit to use it..."

"I want you to stay completely relaxed from this moment on..."

"Completely relaxed, completely relaxed...."

"From the top of your head to the tips of your toes, completely relaxed..."

Deep, deep, deep asleep, deeper, and deeper, and deeper asleep..."

"Completely relaxed, completely relaxed..."

"With every breath that you take, you will get more and more relaxed, completely relaxed, completely relaxed..."

"And now, take in a deep breath, blow it all the way out, and arouse yourself when you want to, feeling..."

"completely relaxed and wide, wide awake, but completely physically and mentally relaxed..."

It will usually take a few moments for the subject to want to open the eyes, because there is such a feeling of peace, tranquility, and serenity, that the subject doesn't want to emerge from the relaxed state. However, there is tingling in the arms and hands, and the eyes just do not want to open. How do we know that there has been a hypnotic state achieved by the subject? During the entire hypnotic session there is a fluttering of the eyelids as though the subject wants to open the eyes, and there will be a redness in the conjunctiva as well as tearing of the eyes. Notice the relaxed state of the individual, and the statement that is so often made is, "I really feel as though I could take a nap right now." "I have never felt this relaxed before."

Another effective method is the hand levitation technique. In this technique, the subject is told to place his hands in his lap, palms down. The subject is told to look at either the right or the left arm and concentrate on it. Tell the subject to notice the feel of his hand.

"Notice the temperature around it..."

"Notice that you can sense the material underneath the hand..."

"The feel of the muscles are quite obvious..."

"As you continue to look at the hand..."

"And concentrate your attention on your hand..."

"you notice a tingling sensation in your hand, and then suddenly your hand starts to grow light..."

"As the lightness enters your hand, you will start to feel drowsy..."

"more and more drowsy, and more and more relaxed..."

"completely relaxed, completely relaxed..."

"Your hand is so light that it feels as though a balloon is tied to your hand..."

"It gets so light that it feels as though your hand will float upward..."

"floating upward, up and up, up and up..."

"Floating upward, floating upward, floating upward..."

"The hand is so light that it wants to keep floating upward..."

"Floating upward..."

(Modify the words so what was first just a visual idea suddenly becomes a reality)

"I want you to notice that your hand is starting to move toward the tip of your nose..."

"Slowly moving, slowly moving, slowly moving..."

"until the tips of your fingers touches the tip of your nose..."

"Slowly moving, slowly moving, slowly moving..."

(The hand begins to move toward the tip of the nose)

"As your hand moves towards your nose, you are getting sleepier, and sleepier, and sleepier..."

"And when you touch the tip of your nose, it will be a signal to fall into a deep and profound sleep..."

"You will look forward to this wonderful experience, and then you will be completely relaxed, completely relaxed..."

"Completely relaxed...completely relaxed...completely relaxed..."

"Deep asleep, deep asleep, deep asleep..."

"You will notice how good you feel..."

"You will look forward to this wonderful experience..."

"You will feel so proud that you have been able to

achieve this depth of relaxation..."

"Continue to relax and go deeper and deeper asleep..."

"Feel how the relaxation goes into the depths of your body..."

"Stay relaxed until you want to take in a real deep breath and arouse yourself when you want to..."

"Staying completely relaxed, completely relaxed, completely relaxed from the top of your head to the tips of your toes..."

I have not elaborated on the above two techniques to have you go out and try to hypnotize another individual. Remember that your subjects have to be selected. You might be able to use hypnotic induction on your friends and relatives, but you do not want to remove symptoms, functional or otherwise without knowing what to do after you have removed the symptom. Functional pain serves a purpose for the individual and at least unconsciously has meaning to him. The removal of such pain will probably lead to the development of some type of new ailment. It is rare that functional pain will be removed without sufficient understanding and insight into the problem by both the hypnotist and the subject. Many subjects cannot be hypnotized in spite of the fact that they consciously attempt to cooperate. Many subjects cannot release their tensions and anxieties so that the hypnotic endeavor can be successful. Hypnotherapy has been found to be a valuable adjunct in the treatment of pain. The response to hypnotherapy varies in relationship to the type of pain, and the underlying factors associated with the pain.

There are many methods of induction of the hypnotic state, and it depends on the versatility of the operator to decide which method is best in his hands. The methods may be authoritarian, permissive, confusion and mechanical technics. All methods involve ideosensory and ideomotor conditioning. All direct methods, such as the eye fixation method which we just reviewed, depend on heaviness of the eyelids, relaxation of the small muscles, with progression towards relaxation of all the larger muscles of the body. The handclasp method may also be used to begin the relaxation state in the subject. The subject is asked to sit comfortably in a chair, and then is asked to clasp his hands tightly, intertwining the fingers very tightly. The conversation goes like this: "You feel your hands begin to tighten, and more tight, feeling pressure on your fingers to close even tighter. And tighter and tighter, so tight that you feel that they are stuck together. Tighter and tighter, tighter and tighter, and so tight that you just can't pull them apart. Your fingers feel like they are one big ball, and you feel a numbness in all of you fingers. As your fingers tighten and tighten, there is a warm feeling in your body, and you start to feel relaxed. So relaxed that you just want to slowly close your eyes and rest. There is such a beautiful feeling throughout your whole body. You are starting to feel relaxed, completely relaxed, completely relaxed, completely relaxed."

Having achieved this feeling of relaxation, you can then proceed with increasing the relaxation throughout the rest of the body. Let the patient keep his hand fixed tightly, since that gives a signal that you are developing relaxation in the subject.

Induction techniques are learned by experience, and if you find one that suits you best, that is the one that you should use. Of course, you may have to vary the semantics relative to each subject, and at times, you will find a subject who cannot be hypnotized by that technique, then you should change just for that individual. Semantics play a great role in hypnosis, and the choice of words many times will serve to induce a state where if the words were changed, the same results might not be obtained. The tone of your voice, and the deflections used can spell success or failure. The higher the pitch of the voice, the less likely it will be that hypnosis will be successful. Don't try to overpower your subject. Speak in a normal tone, and don't try to yell at your subject. The conversation should really be in a monotone, with repetitive stressing of the key words such as "heavy" and "relaxed." This increases relaxation in the subject. Never rush the subject. Once you have given the suggestion, let time elapse before starting in to give further suggestions. Success depends on your ability to work with the subject at that time, evaluating all areas of concern and specifically determining whether or not the subject has responded to what you have suggested.

4

Pain is a sensation which is dependent on the consciousness. It is a well known fact that distraction from attention may exclude from its consciousness many sensations including that of pain. Pain which is perceived is subjective and individual, and it is an emotional as well as a sensory experience. It varies in accordance with the emotional and physical makeup of the individual. Variations in the perception of pain, its minimization, distortion or exaggeration, occur because of associated attitudes and emotions. Words have long been recognized as exerting a tremendous influence on human emotions, and hypnosis as a state of hypersuggestibility provides an excellent means of influencing sensory and perceptive functions. Since pain may originate through the activity of the emotional and intellectual functions of the thalamus and cerebral cortex, hypnosis has been used as a means of achieving relief of this condition. In some cases following complete investigation, although the origin of pain can be properly localized, the cause cannot be determined, nor can the failure to obtain relief be explained. In many individuals the pain cannot be traceable to any causative factor, and personality difficulties with states of tension, anxiety, and other emotional disturbances may become so prominent as to completely mask the primary cause of pain. Because the emotional factor may be so prominent in the patient with pain, hypnosis can be used rather than the usual medical and surgical methods of relief. These methods can be used in the event of failure of the hypnotherapy.

Mesmerism, predecessor of hypnotism, was the first technique used in civilized society for dulling the sense of pain. In the 1780's, Franz Anton Mesmer, a respected German physician, introduced the concept of relieving pain and curing ills through "Animal Magnetism." Theoretically while patients were in Mesmer- induced trances, ailments were drawn from their bodies by a magnetic force. Mesmer had a showman's instinct and succeeded in intriguing-and convincing-numerous would-be skeptics of this novel approach.

In 1821, Joseph Claude Recamier, professor of medicine at the College de France, used mesmerism to induce anesthesia while applying cautery. A few years later, Cloquet performed a painless mastectomy on a mesmerized patient. Subsequently, Mesmerism was employed routinely in hundreds of surgical problems. John Elliotson, physiologist, demonstrated its use in England (1846) with such distinguished observers as Charles Dickens and Thomas Moore. James Esdaile, an English surgeon who was stationed in India, published a report of 300 major surgical procedures and a thousand minor procedures performed using animal magnetism. His report was not recognized in England by the Royal Society of Medicine, and with the advent of chemical anesthesia, hypnosis declined in popularity. James Braid, an English surgeon, was the first to report that hypnosis was a utilization of suggestion, but did not realize that it was the explanation of the underlying process. Charcot, Liebault, and Bernheim had schools in France, but Freud's rejection of hypnosis in favor of his own theories relegated hypnosis back to the stage of amusement and mystery. Mesmerism faded into oblivion in the latter half of the 1880's when other more predictable anesthetic agents were introduced. In later years, however, hypnosis was universally accepted as a means of blunting the edge of pain in patients undergoing surgery. By 1958, the American Medical Association had formally approved the use of hypnosis as a therapeutic tool. During the last 10 years, interest has again been stimulated in England and in this country with research and clinical studies. Today it is accepted as an ethical part of the practice of medicine.

The impressive bewildering character of hypnotic manifestations and the profoundly inexplicable, seemingly miraculous, psychologic effects upon human behavior achieved by the use of hypnosis, have served to bring about contradictory attitudes towards it. The unscientific attitude of superstitious awe, fear, disbelief, and actual hostility have delayed and obstructed the growth of scientific knowledge of hypnosis. If physicians today understood more clearly what hypnosis is and what could be expected of it, then it would be more widely used. Hypnosis is a technique which in skilled hands has very little danger and its application, indications, and contraindications can become a part of the knowledge of the practising physician.

Success in hypnosis depends on establishing selective thinking in a subject with the bypass of the critical factor. It raises the threshold of pain and is the only means of relieving pain which carries no danger to the individual. It is a pleasant experience involving no tension or apprehension, and it can be maintained for a long period of time. Hypnosis places no extra load on the circulatory, respiratory, hepatic, or renal systems. Hypnosis obeys the laws which govern conditioning in general, and suggestion causes new conditioned patterns to be developed. A suggestion is an idea accepted by an individual without resistance or criticism, and upon which he therefore acts. There are as many ways of producing hypnosis as there are hypnotists. Success in hypnotherapy is achieved by being able to match the technique of induction with the subject. Success in hypnotherapy depends on the ability of the individual, and of more importance, on constant practice. It is of utmost importance that the subject believe the competency and integrity of the hypnotist. Under hypnosis there seems to be a dependency of the individual on the hypnotist, and in the hypnotic state the subject tends to carry out the suggestions to please the hypnotist. Under the influence of hypnosis the sensory end organs continue to function but the subject's attitude may be so altered that the pain is no longer experienced in the same way.

Patients with pain need mental and physical therapy more than any other group of patients. Most painful states are not responsive to conservative measures. Drug therapy will usually give relief, particularly opium and its derivatives, but with continued usage the severity of the pain has no relationship to the amount of narcotic necessary to relieve the pain. The reaction of the patient to the pain is dependent on the attitude and mood of the patient. Suggestive therapy has been tried with the use of placebos, but it has been shown that only those of high suggestibility receive benefit from their use. Hypnosis is nothing more than the suggestive placebo effect presented in a specific interpersonal setting.

The mental reaction to pain causes a deterioration of the patient as much as the pain itself does. Under a majority of circumstances pain serves as a protective physiologic sensation evoking bodily reactions which prepare the individual for either fight or flight as a result of the stimuli arising from the surface, or conversely, immobilization, as a result of the stimuli arising in the viscera. However, severe unrelenting pain may be a pathologic process destructive to the individual.

Many times the pain complained of by the patient becomes intractable, that is continuous. It is usually produced by a disease which cannot be treated directly. The application of medical and surgical methods for the relief of pain had its inception early in medical history. Many surgical procedures have been devised for relief of intractable pain; however, these have not been acceptable because of their destructive nature. Such procedures as prefrontal lobotomy, or thalamotomy in nonpsychic individuals will relieve the physical suffering but will also produce a marked blunting of the emotions and of the initiative as well as a lowering of the intelligence. Hypnosis has been suggested as a "psychologic" lobotomy, but hypnosis was tried before and after prefrontal lobotomy, and it did not make the patient more easily hypnotizable as it should if it were a surgical and permanent form of the same state of mind.

Pain causes debilitating states as well as loss of sleep, decrease in appetite, and loss of weight. The use of hypnotherapy for correction of the underlying emotional basis in these patients is advisable, because pain contributes to the perpetuation of the illness. Much of the pain may occur as an excessive reaction to a slight stimulus, or as a guilt complex to a previous situation. The use of suggestive therapy should be attempted early and before addiction to narcotics and alcohol has occurred. It is unnecessary to resort to the use of narcotics in stupefying doses for the relief of such pain when the duration of life may be for only a few months. Relief of the severe pain may be secured at the first session of suggestive therapy, and an attempt is made to secure as deep a relaxation as is possible.

The word, hypnosis, is not used because of the fear the patient has towards the mystery and the unknown. The term, "medical relaxation" is referred to as the method of therapy being used for the relief of pain.

In order to achieve a state of hypnosis, the subject must have the ability to concentrate, the desire to be hypnotized, the ability to take suggestions, and absolute freedom from fear. The presence of fear in the patient is responsible for the inability of the patient to become suggestible. There are certain signs which may be elicited during hypnosis, and if they are present, you can be certain that the subject has entered into a state of hypnosis and is suggestible. These signs are fluttering of the eyelids, injected conjunctiva, tearing of the eyes, physical relaxation, and catalepsy of the limbs. Continued training and education adequately prepares the patient. There are three states which may be reached during a hypnotic session: (1) the light or superficial state in which the subject accepts the suggestion for relief of pain, but it is of no value after the subject is brought out of the state, (2) the deep state in which the posthypnotic suggestions for the relief of pain are successful after the patient has been brought out of the state, and (3) a state in which the subject is so deeply relaxed that there is marked slowing of all organic responses and is of no value because suggestions will not be accepted by the subject.

The depth of hypnosis varies with the experience and ability of the operator. Hypnotic techniques will reduce pain, allay fears, and aid in organ function, but the results are proportional to the depth of hypnosis achieved. Only those subjects who can achieve a deep state can benefit from this therapy. It is in this state that the emotional tensions of the subject can be relieved, and neurotic exaggeration and self-pity can be exchanged for a more constructive and realistic point of view. There is a decrease in the amount of emotional conflict which is present in subjects who have pain.

Hypnoanalysis is attempted with all subjects receiving therapy. The possibility of a traumatic experience entering into the emotional conflict of the subject is always present and should be elicited if possible. When abreaction of some relevant event in the subject's life was indicated, this was discussed while the subject was in the deep state of hypnosis, then brought up to a conscious level and discussed again. The removal of a traumatic experience or guilt complex greatly enhanced the possibility of success of the posthypnotic suggestion.

The advantages of hypnotherapy far outweigh the disadvantages. Drug requirements are lessened and may be removed completely from the subject. The organ dysfunction is corrected, appetite is increased, and depression and fear are removed. The disadvantages should not deter a competent and understanding physician from using hypnotherapy on those subjects who have pain due to inoperable and metastatic carcinoma. The subject needs the support and compassion of the hypnotist, not drug addiction and destructive surgery. Many of the subjects, because of the severity of the pain, do not succeed in using hypnotherapy as a means of relieving pain. Hypnotherapy is time consuming for the practicing physician, and the number of trained physicians in hypnotherapy are still few in number. Other physicians have an aversion to the use of hypnotherapy in the relief of pain, and resort to increasing amounts of narcotics and tranquilizers to make their patients comfortable. Public resentment to the use of hypnosis still persists, and proper education has to be undertaken before it becomes an accepted modality in the practice of medicine. Psychotherapy of any type can be exceedingly dangerous to the subject if the practitioner is incompetent.

CASE REPORTS

The following cases are examples of treatment for painful conditions using hypnotherapy as the method of choice. All patients who received hypnotherapy did not have complete remission from their pain, but the percentage was sufficiently high to continue to use hypnotherapy as the first choice of treatment. Headaches, thoracic myositis, low back pain (pre and post surgical), osteoarthritis, rheumatoid arthritis, and postherpetic neuralgia are examples of the types of pain treated with hypnosis. I studied 178 patients with chronic pain using hypnosis, the results of which were reported in KANSAS MEDICINE (Volume 88, Number 6, June, 1987, Pages 190-192 and 204). The follow-up studies on these patients showed that 78%

were still relieved after 6 months, 47% after one year, 44% after 2 years, and 36.5% of those living after 3 years.

Case 1.

A 32 year-old white female was found to have carcinoma of the cervix. Radiation therapy followed by a total hysterectomy was the treatment of choice. Three years later there was an onset of pain in her left hip and left thigh. A mass was discovered in the left pelvis, and x-rays revealed a metastatic lesion in the left pelvis. She was given irradiation therapy. She had a loss of 22 pounds in weight and was vomiting continuously. She was receiving narcotics and antiemetic medication because of the severe pain and a depressed state. Suggestive therapy was prescribed after consultation with the patient and her physician. The same night, the vomiting ceased, and the patient was mentally improved. No opiates were given that night, and the patient's general condition improved. Further hypnotherapy was given for seven consecutive days, and the patient received no further opiates. The differentiation of anticipation and pain as separate entities, and the use of time distortion was of value in the therapy of this patient. At the end of the fourth day, the patient's appetite was improved, and she was sitting up in a chair. Only an occasional analgetic was needed for a headache. She was dismissed from the hospital with complete freedom from pain in the left hip. She was admitted to the hospital six months later still receiving no opiates although x-rays revealed further metastatic lesions. She had gained sixteen pounds, and she still had a favorable mental outlook. She was released from the hospital after further reinforcement of her hypnotic suggestions for the relief of pain.

Case 2.

A forty-five year-old white male presented himself with symptoms of pain in the left temporal and occipital areas of the head. A diagnosis of herpes zoster was made fifteen months ago, and after the lesions healed, he still had severe excruciating pain in the left C-3 area on his head. His pain had been constant since the disappearance of his lesions, with limitation of motion of the head. Suggestive therapy was started with deep relaxation being achieved at the second session. Time distortion was utilized with some success. Relief of symptoms was obtained through posthypnotic suggestion, and this was reinforced weekly for eight sessions after which he returned for reinforcement at two and six months. No further sessions were necessary in the subsequent months.

Case 3.

A forty-nine year old white female was diagnosed as a diabetic after several admissions to the hospital. She developed acute pain of the left lower extremity primarily centered around the knee. The pain was aggravated by walking, but remained quite severe even though she was given narcotics. A diagnosis was made of diabetic neuropathy of the lower extremity. She continued to have intermittent episodes of severe pain and required narcotics every two to three hours for some relief. Hypnotherapy was started and daily sessions were given for ten days. Relief from pain was noticed after the fourth session and no further opiates were necessary to relieve the pain. Reinforcement was necessary after two weeks and five additional sessions were given. She was again seen for reinforcement of the suggestions in six months, but has had no further incapacitation since that time.

Case 4.

This seventy-eight year old white male was seen because of sudden pain in his left hip which was almost continuous during the day and the night. It interfered with his walking, and started to interfere with his sleep when he changed positions during the night. He consulted an orthopedic surgeon who made a diagnosis of osteoarthritis of the left hip. Surgery with hip replacement was suggested, but the patient did not want to have surgery at this time. He was referred for hypnotherapy, and had five sessions with some relief of the pain, but there was improvement in his walking. He returned after one month for another five sessions, and had relief of his pain, permitting him to sleep uninterrupted during the night.

Migraine headaches are the most frequently complained of symptoms from patients who come to the pain clinic for therapy. Many times all headaches are said to be of the migraine type. Migraine may be said to be a paroxysmal headache which is separated by symptomless free intervals which may be accompanied by nausea, focal cerebral symptoms, unilaterality, and a positive history of migraine headaches in the family. Many times the headache may have visual, motor, or sensory aura accompanying the discomfort. There are also complaints by other patients of tension headaches with migrainous features. These headaches start in the back of the neck and occipital region and may be accompanied by photophobia, nausea, vomiting and pain behind the eyeballs. Functional headaches are usually one-sided in nature, while true organic headaches are usually bilateral in nature.

There may be non-specific tension headaches which can be paroxysmal or chronic in nature. Tension headaches often co-exist with migraine headaches.

Many of these headaches are continuous, and may be caused by allergies. Many of these headaches are predictable in nature, and are dependent on different types of tension states. Atypical facial pain may be present which is a consistent commonly unilateral deep aching or burning pain, usually of many years duration, involving the facial and jaw bones, often extending to the neck, ears, and throat. The characteristic of this type of pain is that it is poorly localized, not conforming to the strict anatomical distribution of any nerve of the head.

In addition, trigeminal neuralgia is a short-lived episode of pain of exceptional severity, which may often recur many times in rapid succession. The pain is restricted to the territory of the trigeminal nerve, and is always unilateral. Individual episodes of pain last typically for a matter of seconds. The episodes are of sudden onset and are separated by pain-free intervals, and may in addition go into remission lasting for several months. Pain is often triggered by innocuous stimuli, such as touching the face, movements, or even gusts of wind applied to the same side.

Cluster headaches are a series of repeated attacks of unilateral pain of extreme severity behind and around one eye, lasting up to twenty minutes. Pain is often radiating to the temple, forehead, cheek, jaw or neck affecting the same side during repeated attacks of the same cluster lasting up to three months. The eye on the affected side becomes blood-shot; profuse lacrimation; congestion of the nostril on the same side; flushing of the face; transient unilateral ptosis (Horner's Syndrome). No visual or sensory symptoms, and nausea and vomiting are rare.

5

Hypnosis has been used for operative procedures with the addition of no chemical anesthetic agents or narcotic sedation which is sufficient to relieve the movement of the patient. Anesthesia may be said to be the loss of sensation with or without the loss of consciousness that can be caused by disease, illness, injury, or chemical agents. To this, of course, must be added psychological means, hypnosis or suggestion. Before the discovery of ether and chloroform, the first attempt to perform surgery with the patient under hypnotic (mesmeric) anesthesia was made by Recamier in 1821. Oudet described the extraction of teeth under magnetic sleep in 1837. John Elliotson, an English surgeon, published in 1843 a book, NUMEROUS CASES OF SURGICAL OPERATIONS WITHOUT PAIN IN THE MESMERIC STATE. He continued publishing THE ZOIST which contained articles of cases of surgical procedures under mesmeric anesthesia from all countries of the world.

On April 4, 1845, James Esdaile performed, in his native hospital in India, his first operation during which the patient was under mesmeric anesthesia. Before leaving India, Esdaile had performed hundreds of painless operations, of which 300 were major procedures and 19 were amputation of the legs. His contribution came at a time when there were no chemical anesthetic agents, and his mortality rate was 50% lower than those of the other surgeons who were performing the same operative procedures. Esdaile claimed that during the operative procedures his patients not only remained quiet, but failed to show the ordinary physiologic signs of pain such as changes in the pulse, dilatation of the pupils, and increase in the respiratory rate, which are characteristic of operations in the nonhypnotic state. The discovery of chloroform and either occurred while Esdaile was in the midst of his surgical practice. As a result, this phase of hypnotism, which might have otherwise seen a great development was destined to become little more than a scientific curiosity.

The literature abounds with references to major and minor surgical procedures carried out under hypnoanesthesia alone or in combination with a narcotic agent, however, anesthesiologists have been working to find more efficient anesthetic agents for the relief of pain. The use of hypnoanesthesia closely approaches the criteria for a perfect anesthetic agent. It is not practical to substitute hypnoanesthesia for chemical anesthesia in every operative case, but there are many who prefer this method to the psychological trauma caused by the chemical agents.

Hypnosis may be defined as an artificially induced state characterized by heightened suggestibility to the hypnotist. The state is usually attained by bodily relaxation accompanied by attention, at the suggestion of the hypnotist, to a narrow range of objects or ideas. A person under hypnosis shows extreme responsiveness to any suggestion made by the hypnotist. It is assumed in hypnosis that the individual's needs, motivation, relevant dynamics, and transference relationships have been sufficiently understood; that there are adequate indications for the employment of hypnosis; and no serious contraindications to its use; that the plan of procedure has been worked out as specifically as possible. Even so, it is advisable to make sure that the individual understands that hypnosis is merely a form of relaxation, that it does not entail surrender of control or responsibility, that it does not make the individual vulnerable to any thoughts or acts contrary to his desires, and that it is being conducted for scientific purposes only.

The individual's motivation, his ability to accept an idea uncritically, and his need to rely upon the prestige of the physican hypnotist are of inestimable value in any form of healing. This is especially important for the induction of a deep hypnotic state. When one wishes to perform major surgery under hypnoanesthesia, it is very important to get the patient to believe the actuality of the hypnotic state, and if this belief is strengthened by the physician's self-assurance, the likelihood of a successful outcome is increased. The patient must be able to accept the physician hypnotist's words as valid descriptions of reality. The physician hypnotist must manipulate his words and the situations in such a way as to lead the subject to believe that the suggestions are literally true statements. These suggestions should be accepted without criticism or analysis. Every patient during the preparatory hypnotic induction sessions must be led to experience the operation with all details and, with this preparation, the patient is protected against any possibility of surprise, fright, and fear.

Many emotional changes accompany anesthesia, and it is well known that stress may produce hypertension, tachycardia, or irregularities of cardiac rhythm. Although every person handles anxiety in his own way, the correct psychologic approach on the part of the anesthesiologist will go a long way toward obtunding psychic trauma and establishing confidence. The usual method of chemical anesthesia requires only a moment or two of reassurance before the anesthetic is started. In the use of hypnoanesthesia, a relatively longer discussion preliminary to the induction is a prerequisite.

The patient who desires to have surgery under hypnoanesthesia must have an intense desire to go through with the procedure. Hypnoanesthesia has been a controversial subject as to its mode of action. It is difficult to say whether painful stimuli to the brain are actually blocked out, or whether the very painful and prolonged stimuli may not produce verbal complaints, facial flinch, withdrawal of part, or changes in respiration only because those functions are at least partially voluntary. Reaction to pain is, among other things, a function of the attitude of the patient. Pain must be considered from both the physiologic and psychologic approach. Pain is a perception and is subject to the influence of associated ideas, apperceptions and fears. Experimentation has shown that the autonomic processes which are characteristic of pain are greatly reduced when the individual is exhibiting hypnotic anesthesia. Electromyographic studies indicate that pain is perceived in the tissues, but during a deep hypnotic state, noxious stimuli do not reach the pain receptors in the higher brain centers. This probably occurs as the result of "snyaptic ablation" (the synapses remain open) in the spinal cord. Apparently the higher cortical centers are not stimulated during a deep state of hypnosis. Hence the vegetative nervous system is able to maintain homeostasis and thus raise the adaptive response of the organism in stress.

Hypnoanesthesia is indicated in (1) cases in which chemical anesthesia and depressants are contraindicated or dangerous because of respiratory or cardiac disease, (2) cases in which the repeated use of anesthetics tend to have a debilitating effect on the patient with an already disturbed physiology, (3) those cases in which it is utilized as the preferred methodology because of the sensitivity of the patient to chemical anesthetic agents, cases in which apprehension and fear of general anesthesia are so great as to interfere with its smooth application or even to result in serious anesthetic risks, and (5) those cases in whom it is desirable to free some of the neuro-physiologic effects of the anesthesia.

Since hypnosis is a quantitative term referring to the relative degree of receptivity to suggestion or command, and has no demonstrable qualitative characteristics as to what proportion of the population can be hypnotized are almost meaningless. Almost all patients can be hypnotized if they so desire. Most normal people can be trained to develop hypnotic anesthesia, but certainly in some people this requires a lot of time. We are dealing with a psychologic technique which involves the total personality of the patient. Hypnosis becomes an especially intense transference relationship. The confidence of the patient in his ability to achieve success and a normal period of conditioning by a trained physician hypnotist assure the surgical team of probable success in the operative procedure. Success also depends on the patient and his attitude towards the approaching surgery. There is no set amount of time for conditioning the patient. Techniques are chosen to suit the individual needs of the patient.

At the first session, the advantages for that patient of the use of hypnoanesthesia in surgery are discussed. Hypnosis is throroughly investigated with the patient so that the apprehension and fear may be removed. Many fear the word "hypnosis" because of the previous knowledge and exposure to the subject by stage and entertainment personalities. Many fear the mystery that has been built up through the years because of misinformation that has been put out on the subject. Hypnosis is a conscious state. The subject is awake at all times. It is a voluntary, consent state, and the subject is not subject to the will of the physician hypnotist. The patient is next conditioned and taken to as deep a state of relaxation as is possible at that time. At times there is difficulty and uncertainty in producing the necessary degree of hypnosis. There are some individuals whose personality make-up is such that it is not wise to increase the transference relationship between patient and the physician hypnotist. The average anesthesiologist has had very little training in the psychodynamics of personality. Such training is essential if one is to be successful with and make proper use of hypnosis, since it is primarily a human situation involving a delicate interplay of human strivings.

Posthypnotic suggestions are then given to the patient to suit the individual needs of each type of operation. Suggestions may be given to the effect that the patient will not feel any pain or discomfort (hypnotic anesthesia). The second suggestion may be that no stimulus, no matter how strong, will disturb him/her. The first suggestion acts to create loss of sensory perception. The latter creates loss of pain perception. Suggestions are also given to produce sedation before and after the surgery. These are effective in lessening the incidences of postoperative atelectasis because suggestion helps the patient to breathe deeply and cough without discomfort if necessary. Hypnosis is also helpful in producing operative amnesia and improving postoperative morale and motivations toward getting well.

In the following sessions, greater depth of hypnosis is secured, and the posthypnotic suggestions are reinforced. While the patient is in the hypnotic state, the entire operative procedure is explained so that familiarity with the procedure is obtained. Each step is explained so that at no time will the patient be threatened with the element of suprise. The patient is tested over the operative site for loss of sensation, and also reinforced through posthypnotic suggestions for maintenance of anesthesia throughout the entire operative procedure. There is the possibility that the patient may be such a good somnabulist that deep relaxation is immediately obtained. Dissociation techniques may also be used as a means of raising the pain threshold. Sometimes posthypnotic suggestions may be given while the patient is in a physiologic state of sleep.

The use of hypnotic techniques will reduce toxicity and lessen the dangers of cardiovascular and cardiorespiratory depression. Hypnoanesthesia offers the greatest benefit and advantages to the patient. There is no loss of reflexes under hypnoanesthesia as there is with deeper planes of surgical anesthesia. There is no need for narcotics for the patient in the postoperative period, since there are no complaints of pain at the operative site, and the ability of the patient to move around further enables a more rapid postoperative recovery. The evidence of postoperative shock and postoperative discomfort may be masked by the posthypnotic suggestions. Although the patient may have no memory of pain following any of the procedures, when rehypnotized at a later date, the site of the pain can usually be recalled and the pain experienced at the time of the operation can be adequately described. Any amnesia present is the result of suggestion and not due to the lack of sensation. This is not the case where chemoanesthesia is used.

To demonstrate postoperatively whether pain was actually perceived although no outward signs of discomfort were visible, or whether the suggestions created a total loss of sensory perception, rehypnotization and recall of the operative procedures should be done together with a running electroencephalogram.

Case reports to illustrate the success of hypnoanesthesia are given in the following pages: (1) debridement of burns with skin grafts, (2) vaginal hysterectomy, (3) bilateral vein ligation and stripping, (4) cesarean section, (5) appendectomy, (6) open heart surgery for closure of atrial septal defect. All of the patients had definite indications for hypnoanesthesia, and all proved to be excellent subjects. An average of five to six sessions, each lasting a minimum of thirty minutes, was necessary to condition the patients properly for their surgical procedure. At no time was there any doubt in the minds of the patients that the operative procedure under hypnoanesthesia would not be successful. Actually, it was the surgeon who were skeptical about the results that would be obtained, however, they were willing to proceed, because of the assurance of the patient and the physician hypnotist. Instructions should be given to the surgeon as well as the operating room personnel as to the choice of words spoken during the procedure.

Instruments and other surgical tools should be handled carefully and not dropped suddenly to make a startling noise. Noise should be kept to a minimum, and extraneous talking and laughter should be held to a minimum. Since hypnoanesthesia is a medical curiosity, there is a tendency to overcrowd the operating suite, and since the patient under hypnosis has increased awareness, this practice should likewise be discouraged.

CASE REPORTS

Case 1.

A 21 year-old female was admitted to the hospital for an elective cesarean section. She had poliomyelitis at the age of three and had residual deformity of atrophy of both legs, scoliosis and kyphosis. Her vital capacity was reduced due to the deformity of the thoracic cage. A spinal fusion had been performed at the age of 8. There was, on X-ray, evidence of fetopelvic disproportion. She was conditioned for hypnoanesthesia at five weekly sessions, a week apart. Posthypnotic suggestions were given for the procedure. Glove anesthesia was obtained at the first session, and then transferred to the abdomen. Skin testing with a surgical towel clip showed complete anesthesia of the abdominal area with no reaction on the part of the patient. Preoperative sedation consisted of Seconal gr. 1 1/2 the night before the surgery, atropine sulfate gr. 1/100, and Thorazine 50 mg., 45 minutes before surgery. Deep relaxation was obtained after the patient was placed on the operating table. Reinforcement of hypnotic anesthesia was accomplished, and a male child was delivered by means of a low flap cesarean section. Pulse and respiration remained within normal ranges, and the blood pressure rose 10 mm.

immediately after the incision was made. Blood pressure then returned to normal and remained normal throughout the operative procedure. Posthypnotic suggestion for discomfort was reinforced before the end of the procedure, and the patient received 25 mg. of Sparine on two separate occasions the afternoon of surgery. Postoperative recovery was uneventful, and the patient was discharged on the 5th postoperative day.

Case 2.

A 54 year-old female entered the hospital for bilateral vein ligation and stripping. She was allergic to barbiturates and was very emotional and apprehensive. She had a mild to moderate hypertension. She was anxious to have the procedure performed under hypnoanesthesia. Four hypnotic sessions were given prior to surgery, and she proved to be an excellent subject for hypno-anesthesia. She was able to enter into a deep relaxed state, and accepted suggestions for anesthesia readily. Skin testing revealed complete absence of sensation to the affected areas after hypnosis was induced. There was no reaction to pain while in the hypnotic state. No preoperative sedation was administered, and she was placed in a deep hypnotic state on the operating table. She was disassociated, and was told to get on an escalator and ride it continuously down into a deep basement until told to stop. Bilateral inguinal incisions were made and ligation of the saphenous vein bilaterally was done. Bilateral stripping of the collateral veins of both legs was completed, and small varices at various locations on the legs were ligated. A small tumor was also excised on the medial aspect of the left leg. The patient got out of her bed and was walking in her room the afternoon of the surgery. No narcotics were necessary for discomfort. The patient was discharged from the hospital in five days.

Case 3.

A 27 year-old female had hypnotherapy for migraine headaches. She developed an uncontrolled menorrhagia and a had a prolapse of the uterus. Two sessions were all that were necessary to produce hypnoanesthesia through suggestion. Skin testing revealed complete anesthesia of the lower portion of the body. Previous experience with saddle block anesthesia for the delivery of her children aided considerably in establishing the loss of sensation. A vaginal hysterectomy was performed under hypnoanesthesia. Preoperative sedation consisted of Seconal grs. 1 1/2. Blood pressure and pulse were normal throughout the operative procedure. Posthypnotic suggestion for the relief of discomfort was given at the end of the procedure, and no postoperative medication was necessary. The patient got out of bed postoperatively in two hours and walked to the bathroom to urinate. She was discharged from the hospital on her fourth postoperative day.

Case 4.

A 28 year-old male received thermal burns covering 80% of his body surface. He had second and third degree burns over his arms, trunk, and lower extremities, and first degree burns of his face. He suffered from severe pain on manipulation of his extremities and movement of his body. His appetite was poor, and because of his critical condition, it was decided to use hypnosis both for psychological and physiological reasons. A tracheotomy was performed because of edema of the larynx and nasopharynx. After the first session, his discomfort disappeared and pain was controlled by posthypnotic suggestion. Repeated debridements and skin grafts were done with the patient using hypnoanesthesia. His general condition improved. Manipulation of his arms and legs was possible without the use of narcotics or general anesthesia. The patient was a good subject and was able to induce self hypnosis on command. There were no complications, and he left the hospital completely recovered.

Case 5.

A 27 year-old female was a previous patient for hypnotherapy for nail biting. She had bleeding from the rectum, and a diagnosis of internal and external hemorrhoids was made. Only two subsequent sessions were necessary to prepare her for hypnoanesthesia. She was told to establish anesthesia simulating a saddle block. Preoperative sedation consisted of Phenergan 50 mg. and atropine sulfate grs. 1/150, 45 minutes before surgery. She was placed in a jackknife position and was given suggestions to enter into a deep relaxed state. She was then told to imagine herself lying on the beach in the sun and listening to music that was being played on the porch of a nearby hotel. She was told to keep time to the music with her finger. An external and internal hemorrhoidectomy was performed, and posthypnotic suggestions were given for the relief of pain around the operative site. The patient was returned to her room in good condition. During the afternoon she complained of pain high up in the rectum, and the rectal plug which was pressing on her fractured coccyx was removed, and posthypnotic suggestion for the relief of that pain was given. The patient made an uneventful recovery.

Case 6.

A patient was referred because of sensitivity to Novocaine, Pontocaine and barbiturates. A diagnosis of chronic appendicitis was made. Hypnoanesthesia was decided to be the anesthesia of choice, and the patient was conditioned in three sessions. He was able to achieve deep relaxation and testing at the operative site with a towel clip elicited no response. The operative procedure was described while the patient was in a deep relaxed state. He entered the hospital, hypnoanesthesia was again established, and an appendectomy was performed through a McBurney incision. Post hypnotic suggestions for the relief of pain post surgery was given at the end of the operative procedure while the patient was still in a deeply relaxed state. He received no narcotics postoperatively, and he left the hospital in four days.

Case 7.

A fifteen year-old female was referred for hypnosis and the possibility of using hypnoanesthesia for open heart surgery. She had a heart murmur, suffered multiple pulmonary infections, and became very tired after an ordinary school day. Cardiac catheterization showed the presence of an atrial septal defect of the heart. Eight sessions of one hour each were necessary to prepare the patient for the operative procedure. She was able to enter into a deep relaxed state and she was given suggestions for hypnoanesthesia. Skin testing revealed anesthesia at the operative site. She entered the hospital, and two more sessions were given on successive days. Preoperative sedation of Phenergan 10 mg., and Elixir Nembutal 50 mg. was administered. Her throat was sprayed with Pontocaine 4% solution. She was told to imagine that she had stepped on to an escalator going downstairs into a basement. 1000 ml. of 5% Dextrose in water was started by intravenous administration. Because hypnotic anesthesia was the agent of choice, after the operative procedure was started, the patient was told to open her eyes. A 6 mm. endotracheal tube was inserted into the trachea, the patient could not speak, but by use of the hands, she was able to calculate arithmetic problems, which she was able to compute. This demonstrated the safety of the heart—lung machine in maintaining cerebral circulation. Immediate consciousness at the end of the procedure showed no complications from the procedure. The heart was open for 14 minutes, and she was on the heart lung machine for 29 minutes. Posthypnotic suggestions for turning, deep breathing and coughing in order to prevent atelectasis were given before terminating the hypnotic state. No narcotics were needed in the immediate postoperative period, and only two injections of Phenergan 25 mg. each necessary postoperatively. There were no postoperative complications, and recovery was uneventful.

There are many advantages to hypnotic anesthesia. It can be terminated instantaneously. There are no depressing physiological effects. It may be continued indefinitely after the operative procedure has been completed. Once hypnotic anesthesia has been obtained, it can be induced at any time. It is a pleasant experience without the nervous tension and apprehension usually associated with chemoanesthesia. There is no extra load on the circulatory, respiratory hepatic or renal systems.

The disadvantages which may influence many physicians from attempting surgical procedures under hypnotic anesthesia should also be mentioned here. One can get overenthusiastic on the subject of hypnosis and try to perform operations under hypnotic anesthesia to inflate one's own ego. Many people cannot enter into a hypnotic state easily. There is an uncertainty in producing the necessary degree of hypnosis. The use of hypnosis without an adequate knowledge of general medical and analytical psychology can be dangerous. Hypnosis is time consuming for the practising physician, and adequately trained physicians are still few in number. Public resentment and prejudice still exists to the use of hypnosis and proper evaluation should be undertaken.

6

Each and every day of the week, there are patients who are seen by their physicians and who are told, "I can't seem to find a thing wrong with you. There is nothing more that I can do with you. You'll just have to live with it." These are the individuals who are really suffering from a state of discomfort which does not permit them to eat or sleep, and usually they become debilitated from a problem that cannot be solved by ordinary medical means. There are many theories as to the mechanisms of chronic pain, but how do we approach the problem?

Because pain is a sensation which is dependent on the consciousness, and is not perceived by anyone other than the individual themselves, nothing shows on the individual to tell the hypnotist that the individual has a headache. Nothing develops on the arms or the shoulders to designate that there is a bursitis, and nothing is present over the hips to designate a condition of arthritis. It is specifically known that pain is a subjective complaint, and being subjective it is very difficult to analyze and treat. However, it is a well-known fact that pain will disappear when attention is distracted. If you have a headache and you get busy talking on the phone, the pain will disappear until after the conversation is over. The headache will then return. The complaint of pain is subjective, and it is emotional. It varies in each and every individual according to his physical and psychological makeup. The first priority to establish is that the pain is real for that individual. The severity of the complaint cannot be minimized, and you can't say, "take two aspirins and call me in the morning." That pain has a cause and a mechanism, and it arises from many different situations, psychological, physical and emotional. But you must honor that patient's complaints of pain. It is easy to say that the individual doesn't look as though he is in pain. If you have never had a pain, congratulations! I hope that you don't ever have to complain of severe pain. Remember one thing. The human mind is subjected to many outside influences in which the individual himself can project the symptom of pain—a symptom that turns out to be a reality to that patient. The patient becomes conditioned to it, and from then on the patient suffers pain that cannot be controlled by conventional means.

As an anesthesiologist I question the use of chemical agents as a means of controlling pain. I have to ask myself over and over again, "What is chronic pain? How do I treat it? Why can't pain be totally relieved by one method as compared to another?" One cannot imagine the pain that is suffered by a patient who comes to you after three laminectomies, the operation of choice in ruptured discs of the vertebral bodies. The pain is still there. The pain is described as being the same that was there before the operations. What about the pain of tic doloreaux (trigeminal neuralgia) after the nerve has been sectioned? The pain is still there. What a descriptive term we are dealing with at this time? The word "pain" is the most descriptive word in the English language. PAIN! PAIN! PAIN! The word denotes suffering, anguish, and discomfort.

Hypnotherapy became popular in the United States in the 1950s. Many individuals who had the qualifications to teach hypnosis, traveled around the country giving three-day courses to physicians, dentists, and psychologists. I had reached the point in my practice of anesthesiology where I needed a challenge other than the administration of anesthetic agents to a surgical patient. Anesthesia was an excellent means of removing pain during a surgical procedure, however, there were other types of pain, other sensations created either organically or psychologically that had to be considered.

As mentioned in the previous chapter, I have used hypnoanesthesia for many surgical procedures. When a patient has an operative procedure without chemical anesthesia, is there pain elicited when the skin incision is made? Is there pain when there is deep dissection of the tissues and the clamping, cutting and cauterization of the affected organs? What is different about these individuals that does not allow them to perceive the sensation of pain? Some might speculate that it is the threshold of pain that holds the answer. Is pain a learned state? Pain is experiential and has to have a prior identification. Through conditioning, we can accept the fact that pain is not perceived. You can feel it if you want to, but the fact remains, why interpret the sensation if not to feel it is for your benefit.

There are many approaches that may be used in

the treatment of pain. Evaluation of the causes of the pain in the patient must be made at the first visit. Several questions have to be asked at that time. Is the pain organic or psychogenic? When did the pain first start? Has it been continuous or intermittent? What treatment has been given for the pain? Does the patient want to have hypnotherapy as a treatment for the relief of pain? Who told the patient about hypnotherapy? Is there a desire or willingness on the part of the patient to use hypnotherapy? Is there a fear of hypnosis shown by the patient? What is the psychologic make up of the patient?

Hypnotherapy in the control of pain is not a simple procedure. The approach in treating the patient must be planned and careful observation must be made of the previous attempts to help the patient overcome the pain. At the present time, we do not know how hypnotherapy works for the relief of pain. What we are seeing is both a psychological as well as physiological change in the patient. One of the most miraculous results that I have seen is the complete relief of pain from a patient who had received thermal injuries of both legs and feet while driving a racing car. An oil line under the the instrument panel ruptured and filled his boots with hot oil. The patient suffered from third degree burns of both legs and feet, dehydration, loss of appetite, and pain. Hypnotherapy was used for pain as well as changing the dressings, and the patient had an uneventful recovery.

The patient is the focus of the treatment. The willingness and desire must be such that there is no doubt in the patient's mind that the pain will be relieved with the use of hypnotherapy. The motivation of the seriously ill patient and the patient who is terminally ill is a factor for success because of the intense desire to overcome the pain caused by the disease and the will to live. Those patients who are negative, hostile, and uncooperative will either fail or the results will be ineffective for the relief of the pain.

Patients who suffer from headaches and general aches present a problem to the practicing physician. Headaches and backaches are the cause of many hours of lost time in industry and business, both because of the numbers of individuals and the stubbornness with which the symptoms persist despite every effort of treatment. The patient who is treated should be made to understand the causative factors for that illness. The patient should be made to develop an insight into that illness and should understand the significance of the problem that causes that illness. The physician should not make light of the patient's complaints, but should show an empathy towards the patient's illness. Patients with long standing symptoms should be shown a way to develop an insight into their problems. Failure to do this can result in lengthy sessions in which very little is accomplished.

In therapy, are direct suggestions better than indirect suggestions for the alleviation of pain? Many hypnotists use hypnoanalysis to probe the unconscious for causes of the pain.

There is disagreement as to whether this approach is necessary in the relief of pain. Hypnosis is just one method of controlling pain and symptom management. In many cases of pain, transference of the symptom to another part of the body is an excellent means of showing the patient the lack of organic basis to the pain. However, we must remember that pain can be a protective mechanism. The patient needs the pain to accomplish a means to an end.

Semantics play a great part in the induction of hypnosis. The hypnotist has the capability of creating an identification between the patient and himself. It is through the voice of the hypnotist that the identification of one's individual self is obtained, and further deepening of the state creates for the patient the reality within the hypnotic state. The way that hypnotic commands are given develop for the patient an emotional level in a hypnotic relationship. Inflections, pauses, tonal quality of the voice are all important parts of the hypnotic session. The hypnotherapist plays a role in which there is an enactment of the level of understanding imparted to the subject. The hypnotic session is between the hypnotist and the patient, and nothing that is said should create a feeling of fright or fight within the patient.

The utilization of posthypnotic suggestions or cues should be used in the relief of painful states. However, the cue is between the hypnotist and the patient, and should not become a universal "gimmick" for all to enjoy. The important thing to remember is that hypnosis is a highly perfected and increased awareness. Everything that is done in the hypnotic state is vastly magnified as compared to what we ordinarily do in everyday living. It is very important to realize the relationship between the hypnotist and the patient when the hypnotist is dealing with pain.

7

To treat pain and painful states with hypnotherapy, it is necessary to understand the approach which is necessary to follow with each individual patient. We must understand that there is not only one method of treatment for pain, and once you have learned the semantics of that technique, it is then used for each and every patient who comes for treatment. Each patient is an individual, and must be treated as an individual. What is the nature of the pain? This question must be answered in detail in order to be able to proceed with the treatment. The most important element in this approach is that you are not just removing a symptom, because if the treatment is for symptomatic relief, the patient will be relieved for a period of time, but will then have the symptom return. You need to evaluate the patient, and as a result you will determine what is the best method to use for the relief of the painful state. The use of hypnosis is based upon knowledge of the individual's emotional situation. Hypnosis is a valuable procedure in giving the patient the ability to be helped in a specific situation that has not been helped with other types of therapy. The individual must be able to be analyzed, and the reasons for the pain brought to the conscious state. Is the pain or painful state, which the individual is having the result of an emotional disturbance, or is it the result of organic distress? The patient has pain, and that pain is real. Any suggestion to the effect that the pain might be the result of psychogenic factors will create a disturbance in the ability of the patient to achieve success in the treatment.

Probably the largest group of patients who come for relief of pain and painful states using hypnotherapy complain of headaches and low back pain. The headaches may be chronic in nature occurring over many years. Backaches and low back pain are usually found in those individuals who have reached the fifth or sixth decade in life. The most difficult symptom to treat is a headache. The location of the headaches varies with each individual. Most prevalent are those headaches whose symptoms begin at the base of the neck and then traverse upward over one side or the other of the head ending usually behind the eyes. Most of these headaches are precipitated by emotional stress or inner conflict. Regardless of the psychological or physical aspect of the condition, the symptom must be treated with suggestive therapy. It is interesting to note, that there is usually relief of the symptoms at the first session. Explanation of the basis of the complaint to the patient seems to serve as a buffer for recalling the symptom at a later date.

Much can be accomplished at the first session, and it is not only the removal of the symptom that impresses the patient, but the significance of the conflicts are brought to the surface and then discussed in order for the patient to realize why the headaches occur and how they can be eliminated. Those patients who have had long standing symptoms of headaches may be difficult to work with, because they usually also present symptoms of inadequacy and emotional instability, and need the headaches to satisfy the poor insight that they might have relative to their condition. However, in some of these patients direct symptom removal does serve a purpose and the symptoms can be relieved for a period of time.

What is the exact nature of hypnosis, and how does it work?

This question has been posed, and there haven't been too many answers to explain the exact nature of the stimuli which affect the body. When we speak of the relief of pain using hypnosis, the pain is not abolished, but the emotional and perceptual reaction to pain is altered. Why is perception to pain readily abolished? Studies have shown that the pain is perceived locally, but it does not reach the pain receptors in the cortex. This may be due to a blocking of the incoming stimuli by distraction of attention during the hypnotic session, and pain is not perceived as pain. The subject is aware of the stimulus, but there is no effect on the subject. Is the symptom removal a satisfactory approach to the relief of pain? Emotional response is also needed to affect a cure; however, the subject has used that pain as a protective mechanism, and as a result looks for the symptom which has served that purpose.

The strength of the interpersonal relationship between the hypnotist and the subject was found to be the responsible factor in success of the treatment by hypnotherapy. The motivation of the subject and the dependence on the hypnotist are essential ingredients for success in suggestion or hypnosis. No one knows at the present time where suggestibility ends and where hypnotizability begins. Hypnosis is difficult to measure, because the results are not listed with respect to the depth of the subject when the experiment was done. Hypnosis is an altered state of awareness on the broad spectrum of what we call consciousness. Most subjects think that they will be in an unconscious state during the hypnotic state, and feel that they have not entered into that state on conclusion of the session. The subject has to be unconscious to their surroundings. What is the sleep that is suggested when an individual enters into a light state of hypnosis? There is a waking hypnotic state, and in that state hypnotic suggestions can be given. Awareness has no relationship to the depth of hypnosis.

There are many cases in which there is failure instead of success in the relief of pain. Many patients cannot be hypnotized because of their resistance to the suggestions offered by the hypnotist. There is a misunderstanding of what hypnosis is all about. The subject has to lose the fear of being hypnotized. The thought that one might lose control, and that this will then be transferred to the hypnotist must be explained at the first session. The most important statement that must be made is that all hypnosis is self hypnosis. No one is able to hypnotize the subject unless there is that desire to be hypnotized. There is only a feeling of relaxation that will be present at the end of the session. One has to be conditioned for the sessions to be conducted by the hypnotist for the relief of symptoms, and very few can achieve the optimum results in only one session.

Little mention will be made here in regards to the similarity of hypnosis and sleep and whether or not there is a change in the brain waves as shown by the encephalogram. Some researchers have made claims that hypnosis is somewhere on a continuum between the sleep and waking states. It seems that hypnosis involves activity at the subcortical level or at some cortical level which is independent of the rest of the cortex during given trance states. It has been shown that suggestions received by the subject will show some changes in response to emotional stress that enters into the state. Many of the subjects will show encephalographic changes in response to the fear and emotional instability which is entered into by the subject at the suggestion of the hypnotist.

When an individual enters a hypnotic state, there is a loss of being in a real world. Even though there is no loss of consciousness, the hypnotic state uses the hypnotist's world of reality as a basis for existence. The subject is giving up to a degree, that control, that for him, determines reality. Reality is suggested from the point of view of the hypnotist, and the hypnotist may enlarge the dimensions of reality that he may organize for the benefit of the subject. The hypnotist should be able to see the relationship which is developing between them, and should realize that this is not something which can be done without resistance. Resistance in hypnosis always exists, although it may not always be recognized. An awareness is the first step in understanding the nature of the hypnotic relationship and may reveal important clues as to how this relationship which has been established can best be used.

Actually, responses due to hypnotic intervention are not necessarily limited to the words or to the direct suggestions that are employed by the hypnotist, but may be intermediate responses determined by the reaction of the individual subject to the meaning of the hypnotic communication.

It can be seen that the simple suggestions that are given are not simple; that the reactions are not based on suggestions alone, but on the reactions and associations made to what the hypnotist is saying. This is particularly true with regard to the induction of hypnosis and some of the problems concerning induction. Some of the subject's reactions to the induction of hypnosis has led to an increased understanding of hypnosis itself. Many subjects tend to equate hypnosis with a deep feeling of dependency, almost to the extent that it creates a problem in maintaining a normal relationship between the hypnotist and the subject. There may be a feeling of personal relationship that can move toward a deeper involvement by the subject which is unknown to the hypnotist. This love relationship tends to satisfy the subject, however, it can create problems as the therapy continues. The subject may handle this relationship with a great deal of personal involvement, however, the hypnotist should be aware of the consequences which may arise if it is allowed to continue. The subject tends to satisfy all of the suggestions of the hypnotist, and it becomes difficult to determine whether the results are real or imaginary on the part of the subject.

In using hypnotherapy for pain relief and pain control, it is very important to understand the emphasis which must be placed on termination of the hypnotic state. The hypnotist should not rush the individual in terminating the trance state. It is difficult to see into the mind of the subject and understand what the mechanism is for the relief of pain. One must speak in terms which will be understood by the subject. It is thought that emphasis must be placed on allowing the individual subject to terminate the trance state, and plenty of time should be allowed for the individual to open their eyes and realize that they have been in a hypnotic trance. The question that should always be asked is,"How do you feel?" This shows an involvement of the hypnotist with the subject, and that there is a concern as to the results which have been gotten as a result. Most of the subjects will want to relax, and take advantage of the state in which they were, and the relaxed state they are in at that time.

Hypnosis in the relief of pain is not new, and the approach must be one of thorough investigation and study of the subject's symptoms. Symptom relief must not be the sole approach to the use of hypnosis. The subject can be temporarily relieved of the symptoms, but this does not help the overall relief of the symptoms. Behavior modification will emerge from a limited perspective of direct suggestion in hypnosis. It is through this organization of behavior that we can better understand the totality of human experience.

8

The individual who is looking for alternatives to traditional medical care has a wide choice of approaches with varying credentials. Some of the methods have well-established records and enjoy high standing within the medical profession. In 1971, when then President Nixon visited China, he became familiar with a practice of medicine that had not been seen in the United States. It was James Reston, a New York Times reporter, who recovering from an appendectomy, was given the choice of relief from pain by the traditional Western methodology of narcotics, or the traditional Chinese method of acupuncture. He chose to use acupuncture, and when he returned to the United States wrote glowing reports on its efficacy. It was this visit that stimulated the medical profession to send scholars to China to study this mode of practice. People in the United States still question the value of acupuncture in the treatment of disease since there has been no particular explanation to the working mechanism of acupuncture that can be understood or replicated in any way.

Today the United States is faced with a difficult decision in the treatment of disease and illness. A branch of classical Chinese medicine has invaded our lives. To most of you who have seen it demonstrated on television, or read about it in journals, it appears to be the panacea for all sickness. Many of us, knowing the pain of arthritis, the loss of hearing, and the ravages of disease which modern American medicine knows no cure, are excited that very soon we will realize the freedom from pain and fear which acupuncture offers. That time is not at hand, although we read about isolated cases in which such cures have been achieved.

As an American physician, I simply cannot afford to ignore the reports of remarkable progress made in the People's Republic of China. Medical men and the public alike have been exposed, and there is a need to know about acupuncture before even knowing that a branch of classical Chinese medicine called Acupuncture existed. Acupuncture offers much in both general medicine and non-chemical anesthesia.

A short time ago, China became accessible to Americans after a lapse of more than two decades. What was the reaction to acupuncture? Three patterns common to laymen and physicians emerged. The first was indifference; the second was skepticism and outright denials with suggestions of fraud, deception or, in some way, political propaganda; the third and minority response ranged from open-minded searching for more facts to the desperate grasping at anything that could possibly bring relief from pain or cure of diseases for which there is currently no hope.

Does Acupuncture really work? In China, Japan,

Taiwan, Soviet Union, Europe, and South America, many patients and physicians are convinced that it does. In the United States, we are strangled by the red tape of politics. At the present time, only a few states have passed laws permitting its use in the practice of medicine.

Pain is so real to almost all of us that it is hard to believe that so much is, as yet, unknown to us about it. No simple neurophysiological explanation accounts satisfactorily for all pain conditions. The way in which some unusual techniques relieve or prevent pain is quite puzzling. One theory that has been expounded by Professor Ronald Melzack of McGill University in Canada is the evidence that there is in the brain and spinal cord a sort of gate mechanism which can be opened, allowing pain impulses to go to the conscious level of perception, or under certain other circumstances, to be closed, preventing the perception of pain. There are instances in Western medical literature in which stimulation applied to parts of the body far removed from the site of pain, resulted in temporary or permanent relief of pain. There is also the theory of the releasing by the brain of endorphins or morphine-like substances which produces a loss of sensation and a dulling of the pain mechanism. Much research lies ahead in establishing a Western neurological basis for acupuncture. It may be a long journey, but the Chinese have taken innumerable steps in 5000 years.

The earliest known text on Chinese medicine and acupuncture dates back to 2600 B.C.E. This textbook is still the main reference of traditional Chinese medical practice. It was through the French Jesuit missionaries that the first accounts of acupuncture reached the West. These early glowing reports were very vague, and it was not until 1928, that a full and accurate account of this curious branch of Chinese medicine became available to European readers. Today, several hundreds of European physicians practice the ancient science and art of acupuncture in conjunction with the art and science of Western medicine.

To the Chinese, acupuncture makes good sense. In the normally healthy organism, they maintained, there is a continuous circulation of energy which is called "Chi." Illness is the result which causes a rearrangement of this circulation. Where energy fails to circulate as it should, vital organs may suffer from a deficiency or a disturbing excess of the life force. Acupuncture is effective because it redirects and normalizes the flow of energy. This is possible because the limbs, trunk, and head are lined with invisible "meridians," related in some way to the various organs of the body. A needle inserted at one of the points on the meridian will exert an influence on the organ related to the meridian on which the point lies. By the introduction of a needle at several carefully selected points, the skilled acupuncturist re-establishes the normal circulation of energy and brings about the return of health to his patient.

To the Chinese, a human being was a living unity, a field for the action and interaction of the invisible forces of life. The harmony of these vital powers within him was revealed by the health of his own body, their disharmony by its disease, their disappearance by its death. So the aim of the Chinese doctor was to correct the imbalance of the vital forces in the body. Once the harmonious interplay of these forces had been restored, the patient himself was able to overcome his weakness.

In the Western world today, the physician tends to picture his patient as a kind of chemical factory or as a none too reliable machine in need of constant repair. The invisible and imponderable powers within him, "spirit," "life forces," "soul," we separate from the physical machine. If they are not mere creatures of our own fancy, they belong to the mysterious and ill-defined provinces of the theologian and the psychiatrist. So when anything goes wrong with any part of the machine, the doctor investigates it as a garage mechanic investigates a badly functioning car. When the fault is found, spare parts are supplied. For example, if the patient is a diabetic, he is given insulin; if he is anemic, he gets iron; if he suffers from some infection, the bacteria which caused the infection are killed off, or he may be immunized against certain infectious diseases, and if his coronary arteries are occluded, he gets a coronary by-pass. The patient is well again until another bolt or nut in the machine needs renewing.

If a doctor thinks in this mechanistic way, he will see a patient as needing the equivalent of fuel, spare parts, lubricants, or emulsifying agents. But in the East, the doctor tends to think of his patient as an organic being with the process of life within him, who can become a harmonious whole in health and vitality, without needing constant replacement for his body. Mind and body form a living unity and cannot be treated as if they were separate. A human being is more than an aggregate of physical substances and chemical processes. Life is something that exists in its own right.

Both the Eastern and Western approaches have their value for the sick patient. We in the West have long taken it for granted that our methods are best, but the ancient wisdom of the East can make a no less important contribution to medicine. In Chinese literature there are descriptions of about one thousand acupuncture points, although there may be even more than that. Books are available that are full of accounts of illnesses that can be cured by stimulation with a needle at one or more points. For example, the point called Bladder 7, near the top of the head with the picturesque name of Penetrating Heaven, has the following effect on: headache, glands swollen in the neck, nose blocked, running nose, swelling of the face, neuralgia of the face, breathlessness, dry mouth, lack of balance, weak eyesight and epileptic-like convulsions.

Since it is so hard to remember the properties of so large a number of acupuncture points, the Chinese classified them into twelve main groups and a few subsidiary ones. All of the acupuncture points are joined by imaginary lines called "meridians." The "meridians" on one side of the body are duplicated by those on the other, just as we have a left as well as a right thumb, but there are two extra meridians which, since they run up the middle of the body cannot be paired.

The number of acupuncture points along each of these meridians vary. The heart meridian, for example, has nine points on each side, while the bladder meridian has sixty-seven. All the acupuncture points on a meridian affect the organ after which they are named. Clearly, this system of classifying a thousand acupuncture points into twelve main meridians and two extra meridians is, in practice, very useful, for if a patient has a disease of the heart, one immediately knows which group (meridian) of acupuncture points to use. One point is usually specific for that type of disease. Heart 7, for example, can cause a slowing of the heart in those individuals with a fast pulse or tachycardia, although Heart 2 or 3 will likewise cause an effect on the heart but will not be as striking as the one first indicated.

How does one attempt to learn all of the acupuncture points? No one really can master all the points for all the diseases that are known. Specific points are listed in an ATLAS FOR ACUPUNCTURE which one uses after determining the disease process which an individual has. The number of treatments required to affect a cure varies considerably. The average patient in China, when seen by an acupuncturist for the first time, does not, as a rule, have merely one disease, but a variety of mild chronic complaints which do not incapacitate him, but simply make life less pleasant. It is a flare-up of these mild chronic complaints that actually brings him to the acupuncturist. All these complaints usually take an average of five treatments to cure. Once a patient has been completely cured of his various ailments, he is then seen by his doctor every six months, and his health will remain satisfactory. The improvement that is noticed during a course of acupuncture treatments does not follow a steady course. The degree of improvement and its duration increases with each treatment until the stage is reached where the improvement persists and becomes a cure at last. Some patients improve rapidly at the beginning of the treatment but may take a long time to achieve that extra little bit that makes a cure. The majority follow an intermediate course. Most often there are ups and downs during the treatment, and there is rarely an absolute steady improvement—nature does not know straight lines. Not infrequently, there is is a setback at some stage of the treatment, which is then overcome by altering the acupuncture points used.

This is the time for Western medicine to accept, as an integral part of the practice of medicine, the art of acupuncture. To try to ignore it, only leads to the practice of what is called, "quackipuncture." Research into the mechanisms by which acupuncture works will take years, and we would still not have the real facts on the subject. A knowledge of medicine is needed to practice acupuncture satisfactorily. It is not only a prerequisite, but it is an important keystone. A physician who has studied physiology and pathology, who knows the causes of diseases and the course of diseases, and who, during his studies and clinical practice, has accumulated a wealth of clinical experience, may tackle a large variety of mild and serious diseases for he knows what to expect if a given organ is stimulated.

The numerous practitioners of acupuncture who are not physicians, who do not know the basic principles of the practice of medicine and who have not studied the acupuncture techniques adequately , unfortunately often achieve results commensurate with their lack of knowledge. Unlike the Chinese who say, "Some people say that one cannot cure chronic diseases, and this is quite untrue. An expert acupuncturist can cure it as easily as taking out a thorn or wiping away snow flakes, or untying a knot or pulling a cork." Even if a disease is of long duration, it can be cured. Those who know acupuncture, know it can be cured.

9

Acupuncture treats disease by puncturing certain "points" of the human body which traverse the main meridians to induce stimulation or sedation. The needles which are used are of different forms, but the one most commonly used is the filiform needle. There are many kinds of filiform needles of different sizes in clinical use. The needle must be stainless steel, and of varying lengths ranging from 0.5 to 5.0 inches. The caliber of the needles which I use in my pain control clinic is 32 guage. The needles must be new and sterilized. They may be disposable, or may be resterilized after each use. The needles must be inspected for hooks on the points or bent areas which will interfere with the insertion of the needles.

The needles are not difficult to insert into the skin of the patient, however, it does take practice to be able to insert the needle without any pain to the patient. The needle is inserted while being rotated, and there may be a slight sensation of pain as the needle pierces the skin. There is little sensation as the needle is introduced further under the skin. Counterpressure in a downward motion may be applied below the point of the needle as it is passed through the skin. The handle of the needle is rotated and pushed so as to cause the needle to penetrate to the desired depth. This method is applicable both for the short and for the long needle.

Pain occuring as the tip of the needle pierces the skin is usually due to unskillful manipulation of the needle and failure to introduce the needle swiftly through the skin. If the center of the penetration of the needle is painful, it may be withdrawn and reinserted into an area just near the previous puncture site.

Certain areas of the skin may be painful due to the condition for which the patient is being treated; however, with practice, the insertion of the needle should not be a problem to the patient. When the needle enters the skin it forms an angle with the skin surface. This may be perpendicular, oblique, or horizontal depending on the location and disease to be treated. On most muscular parts of the body, it is better to insert the needle in a perpendicular direction so as to reach the seat of the acupoint being treated at that time. There is no absolute standard depth for the needle to be placed during acupuncture treatments. Most of the time it depends on the sensation felt by the patient. Generally, the depth is from 0.5-2.0 inches; however, when using acupuncture points traversing the thorax, it is best to insert the needle in a superficial and oblique manner.

In the head and facial regions, the needles are always inserted superficially, obliquely or horizontally, because of the dangers to the opthalmic region.

The general principle is to master the depth precisely when puncturing points close to arteries and veins, particularly if visible to the eye. The physician should be familiar with the regional anatomy in relation to the acupuncture points.

It is not very often that accidents occur, but precautions should be taken to prevent them. As most patients are afraid of needles, the fear should be allayed by the physician the first time that the patient comes for treatment by explaining the procedures of acupuncture. Do not begin until you are sure that the patient will not jump or faint as the needles are being inserted into the skin.

Acupuncture can be traced back to The Yellow Emperor's rule in China. It was he who ordered that a new approach to medicine was necessary to set apart the Chinese approach to therapy, and that the philosophical basis of interpretation was necessary to fully understand the disease processes of the body. The most primitive acupuncture instruments which have been uncovered are stone knives and needles which were used to relieve pain and diseases. With the continued development, the next step was the replacement of the stone instruments with bamboo and bone. In the eleventh century B.C., bronze casting techniques were developed and it became possible to make bronze needles. The use of metal needles became highly significant in the development of treatment using acupuncture.

The earliest medical treatise which is known today was the NEI CHING, the Yellow Emperor's classic of medicine, in which descriptions of acupuncture were written. It is still used as a classic for meridian therapy in China. Channels or meridians were written down in relation to the anatomical and physiological aspects of practice. The understanding of the flow of energy or Chi continued to be studied and began to flourish as a standard of practice distinctly opposite from the thoughts of the Western physicians. During the Cultural Revolution, many relics from the Han Dynasty were excavated, among them acupuncture needles made from silver and gold. Historical information revealed that there was also reference made to the ear, being the place where all channels meet.

The development of coloured diagrams and charts played an important role in promoting the development of acupuncture. In the Han Dynasty, in order to correct discrepancies in the measurement and location of points due to the different body size of patients, the method of measuring a certain part of the body as a unit for measurement, was advocated at this period. The width of the phalangeal joint of the patient's thumb was taken as one unit, and this was used to measure the anatomical locations of the acupuncture points. Physicians and acupuncturists were given formal lectures at the Chinese Medical schools, where experts in the field were the teachers. The standardization of techniques and methodology played an increasing role in the further development of acupuncture.

Treatment by acupuncture began to spread to the Western countries when Jesuit missionaries visited China during the seventeenth century. They returned to France after witnessing Chinese physicians using needles to puncture the skin of patients, and coined the word acupuncture, from the French "pungo," meaning puncture and "accu," meaning skin. Acupuncture is not only broadly practiced in China today, but has been introduced into Japan, Taiwan and the European countries. It also spread to the Near East, and today it is practiced in more than 40 countries of the world. Reciprocally, Western medicine and pharmacology has been introduced into China, and there is an interplay between the two.

Chairman Mao Tsetung and the Communist Party of China have always attached great importance to the development of Chinese medicine. In the days of the Red Army and the resistance against Japan, acupuncture played a vital role in keeping the soldiers and the labouring class in good health. After the founding of the new China in 1949, clinics, research organizations and colleges specializing in Chinese medicine were established using acupuncture and other forms of Chinese medicine such as moxibustion. In 1958, by combining Western and Chinese medicine, acupuncture anesthesia was developed, and is still being used today to a great extent, although the Chinese have the choice of the methodology to be used during the operative procedure.

It is not necessary to accept the Oriental concepts of acupuncture therapy, and the philosophical concepts are too difficult for the Western mind to perceive; therefore, it is of value to have an open mind when studying acupuncture. The Western "show-me" attitude will not increase an understanding of the subject, and as long as you are able to get results, be satisfied and proceed along your own way. The idea of a universal force within the body has been seen in other areas, such as Mesmerism or Animal Magnetism. The life force which creates within us the energy for life can be understood if one understands the souls of the human being. It is not difficult to envision what the Chinese perceived as a life force which provides man with living, and if it is removed, death ensues. This life force is contained within the human body, and moves around in channels similar to the flow of blood through its vessels and capillaries. This network of channels traverse the entire body and are in relationship to the hollow and solid organs of the body, either beginning in the organ or ending in the organ. This is the basis for the anatomical explanation rather than the physiological approach which Western medicine wants to take.

Acupuncture is not to be used by itself as a cureall for the ailments a patient presents. Diagnosis, using laboratory, x-rays, and some psychological understanding of the symptoms presented, will determine if acupuncture therapy will be of value. The Chinese use the symbols of Yin and Yang which are two opposing but interrelating aspects that are always present in the body. They are two opposing forces within the body, magnetic in character, like the two ends of a magnetic bar, one negative and the other positive. The Yin and the Yang are indivisible, and there is always both Yin and Yang. Yin is negative, and Yang is positive, but they are always in direct contact with each other. A balance exists between the Yin and Yang. The organs of the body respond to normal fluctuations and pulsations like the ebb and flow of the tides. No direct scientific evidence is available to prove the existence of Chi, yet this should not be a deterrent to those who want to become involved in the art of acupuncture.

There have been other therapeutic methods which have been developed using acupuncture as a basis. Auriculotherapy is a method to treat disease by puncturing certain areas of the auricle. The relationship of the ear, internal organs, and meridians was recorded more than 2000 years ago. All meridians were thought to traverse the body and meet at a common place in the auricle. Treating disease with ear needling has continued down through the years. Since 1956, auriculotherapy has been used in China, and in particular in France, where more than 200 points have been located through experiments and clinical practice.

It has been noted that when there is disease in the body, the ear reflects this process in various parts of the auricle through discoloration, redness, tenderness, increased reaction to conduction of electrical stimulation, etc. These points serve as stimulation points in the use of auriculotherapy.

The ear is similar to a fetus within the uterus, in an upside-down position, with the neck region downward, and the gluteal region upward. The lobe of the ear corresponds to the facial region, and the antitragus corresponds to the head region. The helix crus corresponds to the diaphragm, and the antihelix corresponds to the spinal column. These points may vary, depending upon the anatomy of the individual and the particular features of the head and neck.

The supra-antihelix crus corresponds to the lower extremities, and the infra-antihelix crus corresponds to the gluteal region. The deltoid fossa corresponds to the genitals, while the scapha corresponds to the upper extremities, and the tragus corresponds to the patient's inner nose, throat, and adrenal gland. The supratragic notch refers to the patient's external ear, and the intertragic notch refers to the patient's endocrine and ovarian organs. The cymba corresponds to the abdominal region including the urinary system, gall bladder, spleen, etc. The cavum conchae corresponds to the chest region, and the region around the helix crus corresponds to the mouth, esophagus, stomach, duodenum, small intestine, appendix, and large intestine. The back of the ear corresponds to the upper and lower back, and groove for lowering blood pressure.

Acupuncture anesthesia, based on acupuncture therapy, which has been used more than 2000 years in China, was developed through the continuous use of acupuncture to relieve pain and promote wellness in the Chinese citizen. There was a combination of traditional Chinese medicine with that of the Western influence in relieving pain and curing illness that resulted in creating this special anesthetic technique which is being used today in many of the hospitals in China. Hundreds of thousands of various kinds of operations have been performed using acupuncture anesthesia, with a success rate of over 80%. Many medical centers have developed different methods of needling, so that many different procedures, including heart operations have been performed in the past few years. Over the past fifteen years, much research work has been done concerning the theory of acupuncture anesthesia, and scientific data has been collected which have further promoted acupuncture anesthesia and the development of medical science.

Acupuncture anesthesia is a new type of anesthesia which may be used in surgery which achieves analgesia through the needling at specific points in the human body. The patient remains conscious throughout the entire procedure, with physiological functions relatively stable throughout the entire operation. It is safe in a wide range of indications. Acupuncture anesthesia is safe to use. It does no harm to the bodily functions, and the technique is simple and the results are predictable. This is very important in surgery, since there is no impairment of kidney function or liver function. Acupuncture does not interfere with the body functions, rather there is a regulation of the physiology of the organs, protecting the body as well as promoting early recovery. Acupuncture anesthesia can be used with old debilitating diseased patients, or the elderly. Post operative complications are few, and recovery is uneventful.

Paul Dudley White, M.D. of Boston, Massachusetts and E. Grey Dimond, M. D. of Columbia, Missouri went over to China as representatives of the United States government and witnessed many operative procedures using acupuncture anesthesia as the sole anesthetic agent. Their reports were documented and written as Supplement Number Nine of the American College of Cardiology Extended Learning, and published in 1972. Many other reports have come out of China since then, establishing the authenticity of the use of acupuncture anesthesia. Its use in procedures such as craniotomies, where the patient's relatively stable condition allows for their speech, and limb movements to readily indicate the functioning of the central and peripheral nervous system so that injury can be avoided during the operation. Acupuncture anesthesia does not readily interfere with normal body function. Blood pressure and pulse remain relatively stable, and there is no postoperative distention or urine retention. The patients can eat and move about almost immediately in the postoperative period. It is relatively simple and not expensive, since it does not require expensive and complicated equipment. It has yet to be developed to that extent in the United States, and will probably never reach the use it has in China.

Since the discovery of acupuncture anesthesia, there have been about half a million cases of various surgical procedures performed. Acupuncture anesthesia is perhaps the most significant discovery in anesthesia since the use of chemical anesthetic agents. One of the most interesting questions to raise is how open chest surgery can be performed without the employment of a positive pressure breathing apparatus. Some explanation is provided by the procedure preparing the patient before the operature, namely, breathing exercises that stress diaphragmatic breathing. Prior to the operation, positive pressure in the pleural space of the lung to be operated on is created by the injection of air. This evidently causes the mediastinum to shift toward the other side. During the operation, the release of pressure on the operated lung following incision produces a sensation of relief to the patient. It is very possible that during the operation the patient may experience some hypoxia and hypercapnia, without positive pressure breathing, but these effects do not seem to be of a sufficient degree to cause alarm or any lasting negative effects.

Acupuncture in China is just another method of treatment for various disease states. Focusing on the treatment of respiratory diseases eventually led to the use of acupuncture anesthesia for surgical procedures. Acupuncture has been used for thousands of years in China, but it was only in 1958 that there was an integration of Western medicine and Chinese traditional medicine. After the cultural revolution, there was a generalized employment of acupuncture anesthesia in open chest and open heart operations with only one or two acupuncture needles inserted into the medial surface of the forearm. This stimulated the research interests of physiologists in China and other parts of the world. It is still in the speculative stage here in the United States, and it is questionable whether or not acupuncture anesthesia can reach the status of other methods of anesthesia for surgical procedures.

10

From the beginning, man has been thought to possess within his body a flow of unknown forces or energy which is responsible for his daily existence. These forces have appeared, at times, to be heavenly, controlling the life of the individual. Investigations have shown nothing to substantiate the claims of these invisible forces in relationship to the very existence of man. The Chinese claimed these invisible forces moved through and resided in definite, although invisible, channels called meridians. This invisible force was labeled as Chi, and was present in living persons. Without this energy life couldn't exist. There were negative and positive poles, and the entire system related to the Yin and Yang which were in close proximity to each other, and could never be separated. Yin and Yang were always in balance, and when there was imbalance, illness occurred. Stimulation of the acupoints during this imbalance brought the Yin and Yang together in harmony again, and the illness was overcome and perfect health was restored.

Whether the meridians are anatomical in concept, or otherwise thought of in physiological or philosophical terms is not necessary to understand acupuncture therapy. Understanding the life force Chi may or may not be necessary to do acupuncture therapy. The fact that this life force resides in the meridians, and the meridians are related to the internal organs of the body and function on a cycle of energy responses, does not necessarily explain the practice of acupuncture. A balance exists between the Yin and Yang, and there exists an approach to the power of these forces in explaining health and disease. We do know that there is a Galvanic response to the acupoints located on the meridian, but the dissection down on a point does not show any type of tissue that may be capable of carrying such a force or current. How then, does the meridian, an invisible channel, transmit the Galvanic response through its acupoints? The mystery remains, and the relationship of the flow of energy to health and disease will continue to be discussed as far as understanding what we are doing to the patient at the time of his illness. What was the beginning of the meridian system? How did the scientists who were instructed by the Yellow Emperor of China come up with this explanation for the practice of traditional Chinese medicine? They discovered that there was a relationship between disease and dysfunction of the body, and that stimulation of these acupoints resulted in the recovery of the patient from disease. These points can be tender, and very sensitive to touch. It is known in traditional Western medicine that certain skin points were indicative of disease, for example McBurney's point in the identification of an acute attack of appendicitis.

When charting these points, one can only pinpoint the acupoints externally, however, the flow of energy enters into the body's cavity and terminates in the organ for which the meridian is named. This is assumed, and has never been verified, except through the continued practice of acupuncture over these many years. In meridian therapy, the body is divided into twelve main meridians which are paired and which continue unbroken throughout the body. Ten of these are named for the hollow and solid organs of the body. Their names are associated with their function, and they relate almost all of the time to that anatomical area of the body. They are: Lung, Spleen, Heart, Kidney, Liver, Small Intestine, Large Intestine, Gallbladder, Stomach, Bladder. In addition there are two unilateral meridians which are called the Vessel of Conception and the Governing Vessel, which are associated with functions rather than organs. These act as reservoirs to store, unite and control Chi. The Tri-Heater meridian deals with the respiratory system in relation to the exchanges of gases, the elimination of waste products from the body, digestive functions, and the genito-urinary function. The Heart Constrictor functions to control the circulation, heart action, and mental processes.

Chi is said to flow through the meridians in a pattern of daily circulation, always in the same direction. This forms a biological clock in which during a 24-hour period, each meridian undergoes a two-hour energy peak, beginning at the Lung meridian at 3 A.M., while at the same time the meridian on the opposite side of the clock is at its lowest energy flow. In addition, the Chinese say that the pulse can be felt, and an interpretation of the energy set in the body can be made.

The twelve channels in their course of circulation

superficially connect with the upper and lower extremities, head and trunk, and internally with the organs. The course of the twelve channels are described as follows:

1. The Lung Meridian—11 acupuncture points

This meridian originates in the middle portion of the body cavity running downward to connect with the large intestine. Turning back, it follows the cardiac orifice, then passes through the diaphragm to enter its main organ—the lung. From the portion between the lung and the throat it comes out transversely. Descending, it runs along the medial aspect of the upper arm and passes in front of the Heart meridian reaching the cubital fossa. From there it runs along the anterior border of the radius on the medial aspect of the forearm and then traverses internally to emerge from the medial side of the tip of the thumb.

Pathological Symptoms: Fullness in the chest, cough, dyspnea, asthma, hemoptysis, sore throat, common cold, chills and aching of the shoulders and back, and pain along the course of this meridian.

2. The Large Intestine Meridian—20 acupuncture points

This meridian starts from the tip of the index finger and runs upwards on the side of the index finger passing through the interspace of the first and second metacarpal bones. From there it goes into the depression between the tendons of the extensor pollicis longus and brevis, then along the antero-lateral aspect of the forearm to the lateral side of the elbow. From there it runs along the anterior border of the lateral side of the upper arm to the highest point of the shoulder and along the anterior border of the acromion up to the 7th cervical vertebra from where it turns downward into the supraclavicular fossa to communicate with the lung. It then passes through the diaphragm and enters the pertaining organ—the large intestine.

Pathological Symptoms: Abdominal pain, diarrhea, constipation, dysentery, sore throat, toothache, serious nasal discharge, epistaxis, pain along the course of the meridian.

3. The Stomach Meridian—45 acupuncture points

This meridian starts lateral to the ala nasi then it ascends to the root of the nose. Descending along the lateral side of the nose, it enters into the upper gum. Emerging and curving around the lips it moves around the middle of the mental labial groove. It then runs along the angle of the jaw going upward in front of the ear and then follows the hairline to reach the forehead. The main flow of energy runs straight downward from the supraclavicular fossa along the mammary line, then descends along the medial side of the umbilicus and enters the lower abdomen. There is a branch which starts at the pylorus, descends inside the abdomen, running downwards to the knee it runs along the antero-lateral aspect of the tibia directly to the dorsum of the foot from where it reaches the lateral side of the tip of the second toe.

Pathological Symptoms: Abdominal distention, edema, vomiting, facial paralysis, sore throat, epistaxis, and pain along the route of this meridian, such as in the chest and knee as well as febrile diseases.

4. The Spleen Meridian—20 acupuncture points

This meridian originates in the medial side of the great toe, and from there it runs along the junction of skin of the foot and sole and ascends in front of the medial malleolus up to the leg. It continues along the posterior surface of the tibia, medial aspect of the leg, then it passes through the anterior medial aspect of the knee and thigh, and enters the abdominal cavity further up and goes to the spleen, its pertaining organ, and communicates with the stomach. From there it passes through the diaphragm and ascending along the esophagus reaches both sides of the root of the tongue and spreads over its lower surface.

Pathological Symptoms: Stiffness and pain in the tongue, gastric pain, abdominal distention, vomiting, jaundice, general weakness and heaviness of the body, and pain and swelling along the course of the meridian.

5. The Heart Meridian—9 acupuncture points

This channel runs traversely from the heart to the lung, then descends emerging from the axilla, passing along the posterior border of the medial aspect of the upper arm behind the Lung meridian. It then continues down to the cubital fossa, then along the posterior border of the medial aspect of the forearm to the capitate bone proximal to the palm then via the palm along the medial side of the little finger to its tip.

Pathological Symptoms: Dryness of the throat, pain in the cardiac or hypochrondriac region, thirst, jaundice, increase in the temperature of the palm, and pain along the course of this meridian.

6. The Small Intestine Meridian—19 acupuncture points

This meridian starts from the ulnar side of the tip of the little finger, follows the ulnar side of the palm to the wrist and emerges from the styloid process of the ulna. From there it passes straight upward along the posterior aspect of the forearm, passes between the olecranon of the ulna and medial epicondyle of the humerus and runs along the posterior border of the lateral aspect of the upper arm to the shoulder joint. It then circles around the shoulder, turning downward into the supraclavicular fossa where it joins the heart. From there it descends along the esophagus, passes through the diaphragm to the stomach, finally entering its pertaining organ, the small intestine.

Pathological Symptoms: Pain in the lower abdomen, deafness, jaundice, swelling of the cheek, sore throat and pain along the course of this meridian.

7. The Urinary Bladder Meridian—52 acupuncture points

This meridian commences at the inner canthus of the eye ascends to the forehead and joins its symmetrical meridian at the vertex, where the original meridian enters into and communicates with the brain from the vertex, and then re-emerges, bifurcating at the back of the neck and running downward along the medial side of the scapula, then parallel to the vertebral column to the lumbar region where it enters into the body cavity through the paravertebral muscles, communicating with the kidney and finally joining its pertaining organ, the urinary bladder. It continues down through the gluteal muscles and ends in the popliteal fossa.

Pathological Symptoms: Retention of urine, eneuresis, headache, eye diseases, pain along the course of this meridian, such as in the back, neck, lumbar region and lower extremities.

8. The Kidney Meridian—27 acupuncture points

This meridian starts from the inferior aspect of the little toe, running towards the sole, emerging from the inferior aspect of the tuberosity of the navicular bone and running behind the medial malleolus, it enters into the heel. Then it descends along the medial side of the leg to the medial side of the popliteal fossa, advancing further along the medio-posterior aspect of the thigh towards the vertebral column to enter its pertaining organ, the kidney, to communicate with the urinary bladder. Re-emerging from the kidney, running straight upward and passing through the liver and diaphragm it enters the lung, runs along the esophagus and terminates at the root of the tongue.

Pathological Symptoms: Hemoptysis, dyspnea, dryness of the tongue, sore throat, lumbago, edema, constipation, diarrhea, motor impairment and muscular atrophy of the lower extremities, increase in temperature of the sole of the foot, and pain along the course of the meridian.

9. The Gall Bladder Meridian—44 acupuncture points

This meridian starts from the outer canthus ascends to the corner of the forehead, curves downward to the retro-auricular area and runs along the side of the neck to the shoulder. Turning backward, this meridian runs posteriorly and downward to the supraclavicular fossa. From the supraclavicular fossa it runs downward, passes in front of the axilla and along the lateral aspect of the chest. Then it descends along the lateral aspect of the thigh to the lateral side of the knee, from where it continues downward, passes through the anterior aspect of the fibula directly to its lower end, then runs further downward and anteriorly to the external malleolus, along the dorsum of the foot, terminating at the lateral side of the tip of the 4th toe.

Pathological Symptoms: Bitter taste in the mouth, dizziness, malaria, headache, pain in the submaxillary region, pain in the outer canthus, deafness, tinnitus, and pain along the course of this meridian.

10. The Liver Meridian—14 acupuncture points

This meridian starts from the dorsal region of the great toe, passes the dorsum of the foot one inch in front of the medial malleolus. From there it ascends 8 inches above the medial malleolus further ascending along the medial side of the knee and thigh to the pubic region where it curves around the external genitalia to the lower abdomen. From there, the meridian runs upward, encircles the stomach and enters the pertaining organ, the liver, to communicate with the gall bladder. Further upward it passes through the diaphragm, the costal and hypochondriac region, ascends along the posterior aspect of the throat to the nasopharynx and connect with the eye, then emerges at the forehead to end at the vertex.

Pathological Symptoms: Lumbago, fullness of chest, vomiting, eneuresis, retention of urine, hernia, and pain in the lower abdomen.

11. The Governing Vessel—28 acupuncture points

This meridian starts in the pelvic cavity, descends and emerges at the perineum, passing through the tip of the coccyx and ascending along the middle of the spinal column to communicate with the kidney in the lumbar region. Then it ascends to the brain reaching the vertex, winding in the midline of the forehead to the columella of the nose to descend to the upper lip where it terminates.

Pathological Symptoms: Febrile diseases, mental disorders, stiffness and pain in the spinal column, opisthotonos, etc.

12. Vessel of Conception—24 acupuncture points

This meridian starts from the pelvic cavity and emerges at the perineum, then runs anteriorly across the pubic region and ascends along the midline of the abdomen through the chest up to the throat and mandible, curving around the lips.

Pathological Symptoms: Hernia, leukorrhea, cough and dyspnea, diseases of the urogenital system.

As mentioned above, the meridians communicate with the internal organs interiorly, and with the extremities exteriorly, performing the physiological function of the circulating Chi and connecting the superficial and interior portions of the human body, thus protecting it from attacks of etiological factors. For example, when the human body is attacked by exogenous factors, or other circumstances cause an imbalance of the Chi, corresponding pathological changes will naturally occur in the meridians and their pertaining organs. Generally speaking, exogenous diseases are always carried to the internal portion of the body from the external, and it is the meridians that are always attacked first by the exogenous factors. On the other hand, diseases caused by exogenous factors usually first occur in the internal organs and finally in the meridians. Therefore it is easy to see that pathology in the meridians means derangement of the function of the meridians and their effect on the viscera, and the effect of the pathological changes of the internal organs on the meridians.

Each of the meridians , either Yin or Yang, pertain to the internal viscera. Those that pertain to the solid organs (heart, lung, spleen, kidney and liver are called the Yin meridians, and those that pertain to the hollow organs (large and small intestines, stomach, bladder, and gall and urinary bladders) are called the Yang meridians. Each of the Yin meridians couples with a Yang meridian. The Yin meridians run along the lateral aspect, being opposite to each other. In circulation, the Yin meridians flow into the solid organs, and communicate with the hollow organs, while the Yang meridians flow into the hollow organs and communicate with the solid organs, and so six pairs of interior-exterior related channels are formed.

11

In learning the acupuncture points, it is necessary to know the exact locations of the points. There are various acupuncture therapy machines that incorporate an instrument for locating the points via measurement of a galvanometer. The probe is used to find the exact location of the point, and when the tip is pressed down on the location, there is a deflection of the needle of the galvanometer. The location which shows the greatest deflection of the needle is the point on the meridian identified. It takes constant investigation and practice to learn the points of the various meridians. The majority of the points are identified in relation to anatomical structures which can be identified on the body. There are identifiable landmarks that will be established, so that each and every acupuncture point is measured in exactly the same way. For example, the distance between the two creases marking the joints of the distal and middle phalanges of the middle finger is one inch. The breadth of the first joint of the thumb is one inch. The breadth of the four fingers close together at the second joint of the index finger is calculated as three inches. These measurements are simple to apply in learning the acupuncture points.

The forearm of the patient from the transverse crease of the wrist to the cubital fossa is measured as 12 inches. These methods of measurement can be applied accurately to a child as well as to an adult, patients of various body build, whether obese or thin, tall or short, as the length of an inch is variable accordingly. Examples of the various measurements of the body are as follows:

1. Anterior hairline to posterior hairline = 12 inches
2. Posterior hairline to the process of the 7th cervical vertebrae = 3 inches
3. Hairline between the two temporal regions = 9 inches
4. Distance between the two nipples = 8 inches
5. From the end of the sternum to the umbilicus = 8 inches
6. Center of the umbilicus to upper border of symphysis pubis = 5 inches
7. Upper level of the greater trochanter to the middle of patella = 19 inches
8. Middle of patella to tip of lateral malleolus = 16 inches
9. Middle condyle of the tibia to the tip of the medial malleolus = 13 inches

Points can be located according to anatomical landmarks. The sense organs can be taken as landmarks in locating points on the head. For the back, the process of the vertebral spines, the scapula (the tip of the scapular spine is level with the 3rd thoracic vertebral spine, the ribs, and the iliac crest which is on a level with the 4th lumbar vertebra serve as landmarks. Serving as landmarks for the chest and abdomen are the nipples, umbilicus, sternum, pubic bone, etc., and for the four limbs, the joints and condyles may be taken as landmarks.

Let us now study the landmarks of the various meridian beginning with the Lung meridian which has 11 acupuncture points. It would be wise to copy down the landmarks and have them available to mark on a picture of the human skeleton, both the anterior and posterior views. In giving the indications, only those points which are related to the relief of pain will be listed. Other indications may be found in any standard textbook of acupuncture therapy.

The Lung Meridian

1. Lu. 1 -

Location: On the lateral aspect of the chest, in the interspace of the 1st and 2nd ribs, 6 in. lateral to the midline of the chest.

Indications: Pain in chest, shoulder and back pain

2. Lu. 2 -

Location: Below the acromial extremity of the clavicle in the depression lateral to the triangle of the pectoralis muscle, 6 in. lateral to the midline of the chest.

Indications: Pain in chest, pain in shoulder and chest.

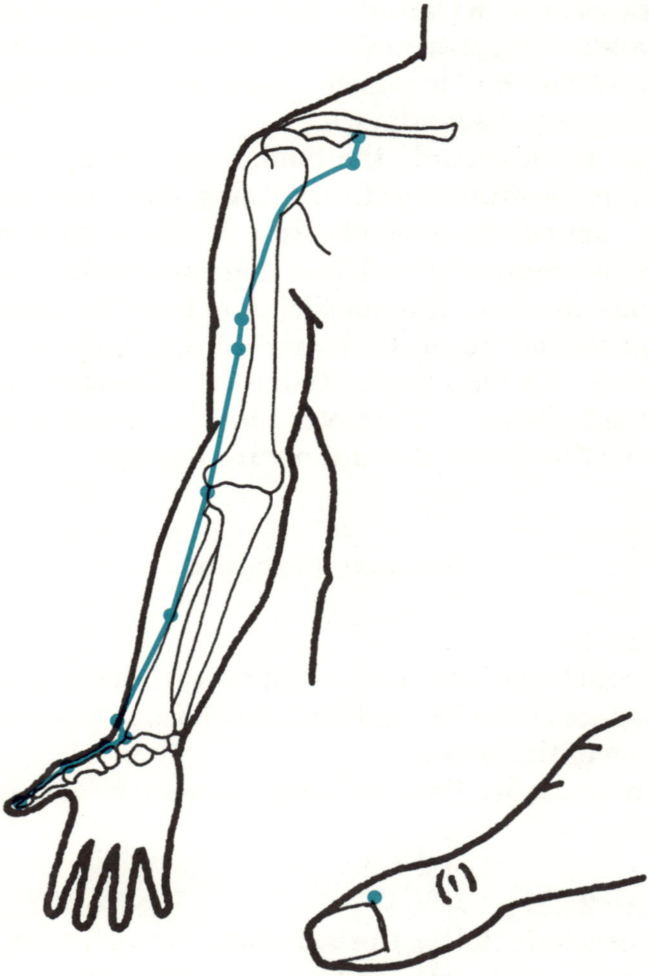

The Lung Meridian

3. Lu. 3 -

Location: On the medial aspect of the upper arm, 3 in. below the anterior axillary fold, on the radial side of biceps radialis muscle , 6 in. above Lu. 5.

Indications: Pain in the medial aspect of the upper arm.

4. Lu. 4 -

Location: On the medial side of the upper arm, antero-lateral to the humerus, on the radial side of the biceps bracialis, 1 in. below Lu. 3.

Indications: Pain in the chest, pain in the medial aspect of the upper arm.

5. Lu. 5 -

Location: In the cubital crease, on the radial side of the tendon of m. brachialis biceps, flex elbow slightly to locate the point.

Indications: Pain and swelling in the elbow and the arm.

6. Lu. 6 -

Location: On the radial aspect of the arm, 7 in. above the wrist crease.

Indications: Pain and impairment of the elbow and arm.

7. Lu. 7 -

Location: Above the styloid process of the radius, 1.5 in. above the transverse crease of the wrist.

Indications: Headaches, stiffness of the neck, facial paralysis.

8. Lu. 8 -

Location: 1 inch above the transverse fold of the wrist, in the medial aspect of the styloid process of the

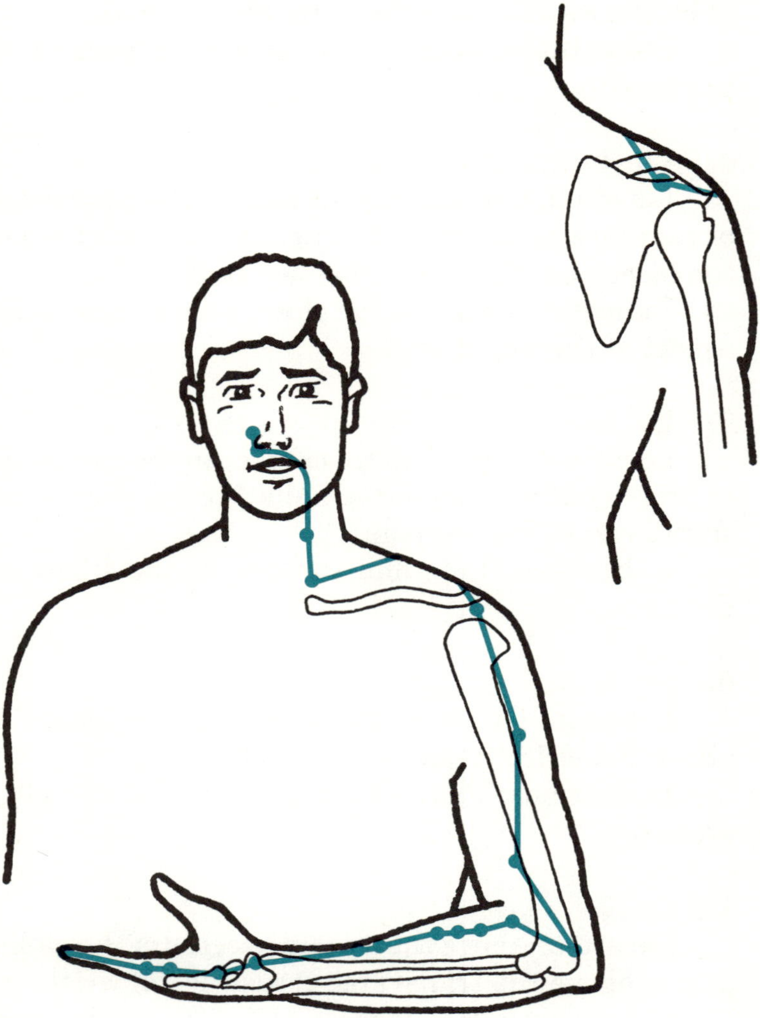

The Large Intestine Meridian

radius.

Indications: Pain in the chest, sore throat, pain in the wrist and hand.

9. Lu. 9 -

Location: On the palmar surface, at the tip of the transverse crease of the wrist, in the depression on the radial side of the radial artery.

Indications: Chest pain, asthma, pain in the back and shoulders.

10. Lu. 10 -

Location: On the palmar surface, in the middle of the 1st metacarpal bone.

Indications: Asthma, sore throat.

11. Lu. 11 -

Location: On the radial side of the thumb, about 0.1 in. posteriorly to the corner of the nail.

Indications: Respiratory failure, epilepsy, tonsillitis.

The Large Intestine Meridian

1. L.I. 1 -

Location: On the radial side of the index finger, 0.1 in. posterior to the corner of the nail.

Indications: Pain and swelling in the throat and pharynx.

2. L.I. 2 -

Location: In the depression distal to the 2nd metacarpo-phalangeal joint on the radial side. Clench fist to locate the point.

Indications: Toothache, sore throat, shoulder and

back pain, facial paralysis.

3. L.I. 3 -

Location: On the radial side of the index finger in a depression proximal to the head of the second metacarpal bone.

Indications: Toothache, sore throat, trigeminal neuralgia, swelling of fingers and back of the hand.

4. L.I. 4 -

Location: On the middle of the 2nd metacarpal bone, on the radial aspect. It can also be found as the highest point of the muscle when the thumb and index finger are brought together, or stretch the thumb and index finger. The point is mid-distant on a line between the junction and the 1st and 2nd metacarpal bones and the border of the web, slightly towards the 2nd metacarpal bone.

Indications: Headache, toothache, pain and paralysis of the upper extremities, arthritis of the mandible.

5. L.I. 5 -

Location: On the radial side of the back of the wrist. When the thumb is tilted upward, it is in the hollow between the tendons of m. extensor pollicis brevis and longus.

Indications: Headache, tinnitus, toothache, pain in the wrist and hand.

6. L.I. 6 -

Location: 3 inches above L.I. 5.

Indications: Tonsillitis, facial paralysis, pain in the forearm, edema.

7. L.I. 7 -

Location: 5 in. above L.I. 5 on a line connecting L.I. 5 and L.I. 11.

Indications: Stomatits, parotitis, aching of the shoulder and arm.

8. L.I. 8 -

Location: 4 in. below L.I. 11.

Indications: Pain in the elbow and arm, abdominal pain, mastitis.

9. L.I. 9 -

Location: 3 in. below L.I. 11.

Indications: Aching of shoulder and back, tingling and numbness of upper extremities, abdominal pain.

10. L.I. 10 -

Location: On a line connecting L.I. 5 and L.I. 11, 2 in. directly below the latter.

Indications: Pain in the shoulder and arm, tremor, hemiplegia.

11. L.I. 11 -

Location: In the depression at the lateral end of the transverse cubital crease. Midway between Lu. 5 and the lateral epicondyle of the humerus, when the elbow is half flexed.

Indications: Pain in the shoulder and arm, paralysis of the upper extremities, neurodermatitis, disorder of the cubital joint and its surrounding tissue.

12. L.I. 12 -

Location: Superior to the lateral epicondyle of the humerus, on the lateral border of the humerus.

Indications: Pain, contracture and numbness in the elbow and arm.

13. L.I. 13 -

Location: On the antero-medial border of the humerus, 3 in. above the elbow crease.

Indications: Peritonitis, pain in the elbow and arm.

14. L.I. 14 -

Location: At the lower end of the deltoid muscle of the humerus, in line with L.I. 11 and L.I. 15.

Indications: Pain and impairment of movement of elbow and arm, disorder of the shoulder joint and its surrounding soft tissue.

15. L.I. 15 -

Location: (a) At the anterior and inferior border of the acromio-clavicular joint, inferior to the acromion, when the arm is in adduction. (b) The point is in the depression of the acromion when the arm is in full abduction.

Indications: Pain and impairment of movement of elbow and arm, disorder of the shoulder joint and its surrounding soft tissue.

16. L.I. 16 -

Location: In the depression between the acromio-clavicular extremity and the spine of the acapula.

Indications: Pain in the back, shoulder and upper extremities.

17. L.I. 17 -

Location: About 1 in. below L.I. 18, at the posterior border of the sterno-cleido mastoid muscle, when patient sits straight with head tilted back.

Indications: Sore throat, tonsillitis.

18. L.I. 18 -
Location: 3 in. lateral to the thyroid cartilage, between the sternal head and the clavicular head of the sterno-cleido-mastoid muscle.
Indications: Cough, sore throat.

19. L.I. 19 -
Location: 0.5 in. lateral to the midpoint of the upper lip.
Indications: Epistaxis, nasal obstruction, facial paralysis.

20. L.I. 20 -
Location: Between the naso-labial groove and the midpoint of the outer border of the nasal ala.
Indications: Rhinitis, sinusitis, facial paralysis.

The Stomach Meridian

The Stomach meridian contain 45 acupuncture points. They are as follows:

1. St. 1 -
Location: Between the eyeball and the midpoint of the infra-orbital ridge.
Indications: Conjunctivitis, thermal burns.

2. St. 2 -
Location: 0.7 in. below St. 1, in the depression at the infra-orbital foramen.
Indications: Headache, twitching of the eyelids, facial paralysis.

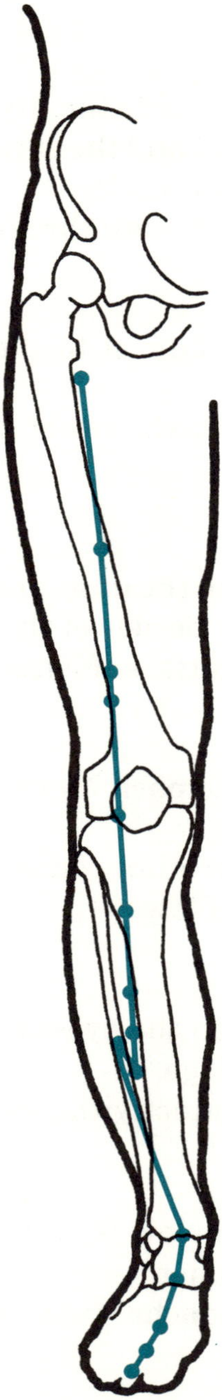

The Stomach Meridian

3. St. 3 -

Location: Directly below St. 2 at the level of the lower end of the ala nasi, lateral to the naso-labial groove.

Indications: Toothache, pain and swelling of the lips and cheeks.

4. St. 4 -

Location: 0.4 in. lateral to the corner of the mouth.

Indications: Trigeminal neuralgia, salivation.

5. St. 5 -

Location: Anterior to the angle of the jaw, at the lower border of m. masseter where the artery of the mandibular groove can be palpated.

Indications: Toothache, parotitis.

6. St. 6 -

Location: Anterior and superior to the angle of the jaw at the prominence of the masseter muscle when the jaw is shut tight.

Indications: Toothache, spasm of the masseter muscle.

7. St. 7 -

Location: In the depression at the lower border of the zygomatic arch, anterior to the condyloid process of the mandible.

Indications: Trigeminal neuralgia, toothache, mandibular arthritis.

8. St. 8 -

Location: 0.5 in. within the anterior hairline at the corner of the forehead.

Indications: Migraine, lacrimation.

9. St. 9 -

Location: Posterior to the common carotid artery on the anterior border of the sterno-cleido-mastoid muscle, lateral to the thyroid cartilage.

Indications: Hypertension, sore throat, asthma.

10. St. 10 -

Location: On the anterior border of the sterno-cleido-mastoid muscle, midway between St. 9 and St. 11.

Indications: Sore throat, asthma.

11. St. 11 -

Location: Directly below St. 9 on the superior border of the clavicle.

Indications: Sore throat, dyspnea, stiff neck.

12. St. 12 -

Location: In the middle of the supraclavicular fossa, on the mammillary line.

Indications: Sore throat, asthma, pleuritis, costal neuralgia.

13. St. 13 -

Location: Below the midpoint of the clavicle.

Indications: Asthma, bronchitis, chest and back pain, hiccough, dyspnea.

14. St. 14 -

Location: In the 1st intercostal interspace.

Indications: Bronchitis, distention and pain in the chest and hypochrondriac region.

15. St. 15 -

Location: In the 2nd interspace.

Indications: Bronchitis, distention and pain in

the chest and costal region, asthma.

16. St. 16 -

Location: In the 3rd interspace.

Indications: Cough, asthma, pain in the hyperchrondiac region, mastitis.

17. St. 17 -

Location: In the center of the nipple, in the 4th costal interspace, midline of the clavicle.

Indications: (NOTE) This point only serves as a marking for transverse measurement in locating the points on the chest and abdomen. The distance between the two nipples is 8 in.

18. St. 18 -

Location: Directly below the nipple in the depression of the mammary groove, in the 5th intercostal space.

Indications: Mastitis, chest pain.

19. St. 19 -

Location: 6 in. above the umbilicus.

Indications: Intercostal neuralgia.

20. St. 20 -

Location: 5 in. above the umbilicus.

Indications: Acute and chronic gastritis, pain and spasm of the rectus abdominis muscle.

21. St. 21 -

Location: 4 in. above the umbilicus.

Indications: Gastric or duodenal ulcer, acute or chronic gastritis, gastric neurosis.

22. St. 22 -
Location: 3 in above the umbilicus.
Indications: Abdominal pain or distention, anorexia, edema, diarrhea.

23. St. 23 -
Location: 2 in. above the umbilicus.
Indications: Hernia, eneuresis, mental disorder.

24. St. 24 -
Location: 1 in. above umbilicus.
Indications: Nausea and vomiting, mental disorder.

25. St. 25 -
Location: 2 in. lateral to the umbilicus.
Indications: Acute and chronic gastro-enteritis, dysentery, constipation, appendicitis, acute intestinal obstruction.

26. St. 26 -
Location: 1 in. below umbilicus.
Indications: Abdominal pain, menorrhagia.

27. St. 27 -
Location: 2 in. below umbilicus.
Indications: Cystitis, abdominal pain.

28. St. 28 -
Location: 3 in. below umbilicus.
Indications: Nephritis, cystitis, retention of urine.

29. St. 29 -
Location: 4 inches below umbilicus.
Indications: Amenorrhea, prolapse of uterus, acute epididymitis, chronic pelvic inflammation, hernia.

30. St. 30 -

Location: 5 in. below umbilicus.

Indications: urogenital diseases, hernia.

31. St. 31 -

Location: Directly below the anterior superior iliac spine, in a line level with the lower border of the symphysis pubis.

Indications: Paralysis of lower extremities, hemiplegia, rheumatism.

32. St. 32 -

Location: 6 in. above the border of the patella, or cover knee-cap with hand, the middle of the 1st wrist crease on middle of knee, fingers close together. The point is where the middle finger rests.

Indications: Pain, paralysis of lower extremities, hemiplegia.

33. St. 33 -

Location: In a depression 3 in. above the superolateral border of the patella.

Indications: Aching of the knee joint and leg.

34. St. 34 -

Location: In a depression 2 in. above the superolateral edge of the patella.

Indications: mastitis, disorders of the knee joint and its surrounding soft tissue.

35. St. 35 -

Location: Ask the patient to bend the knee, The point is in the depression just below the patella, lateral to the patellar ligament.

Indications: Arthritis of the knee joint.

36. St. 36 -

Location: 3 in. below St. 35, one finger breadth from the anterior crest of the tibia.

Indications: Nausea and vomiting, abdominal distention, constipation, and diseases of the digestive tract.

37. St. 37 -

Location: 6 in. below St. 35, one finger breadth from the anterior crest of the tibia.

Indications: Abdominal pain, diarrhea, appendicitis, paralysis of the lower extremities.

38. St. 38 -

Location: 8 inches below the knee, 2 in. below St. 37.

Indications: Paralysis or aching of the lower extremities, gastric or abdominal pain, peri-arthritis of the shoulder.

39. St. 39 -

Location: 3 in. below St. 37.

Indications: Abdominal pain, paralysis of the lower extremities.

40. St. 40 -

Location: 8 in. below the knee; one finger breadth lateral to St. 38.

Indications: Cough, dizziness and vertigo, numbness of the lower extremities, hemiplegia.

41. St. 41 -

Location: On the midpoint of the dorsum of the foot at the transverse malleolus crease, between the tendons of the extensor digitorum longus muscle and hallucis longus muscle.

Indications: Paralysis of lower extremities, disorders of the malleolar joint and its surrounding tissue.

42. St. 42 -

Location: 1.5 in. distal to St. 41, at the highest point of the dorsum of the foot, where the artery can be palpated.

Indications: Pain in the dorsum of the foot, toothache, epilepsy.

43. St. 43 -

Location: In the depression distal to the junction of the 2nd and 3rd metatarsal bones.

Indications: Facial swelling, abdominal pain, pain and swelling of the dorsum of the foot, tonsillitis.

44. St. 44 -

Location: 0.5 in. proximal to the web margin between the 2nd and 3rd toes.

Indications: Headache, tonsillitis, toothache.

45. St. 45 -

Location: On the lateral side of the tip of the 2nd toe, 0.1 in posterior to the corner of the nail.

Indications: Febrile diseases, dream disturbed sleep, epilepsy.

The Pericardium Meridian

The Pericardium meridian has nine acupuncture points: They are as follows:

1. P. 1 -

Location: 1 in. lateral to the nipple in the 4th intercostal space.

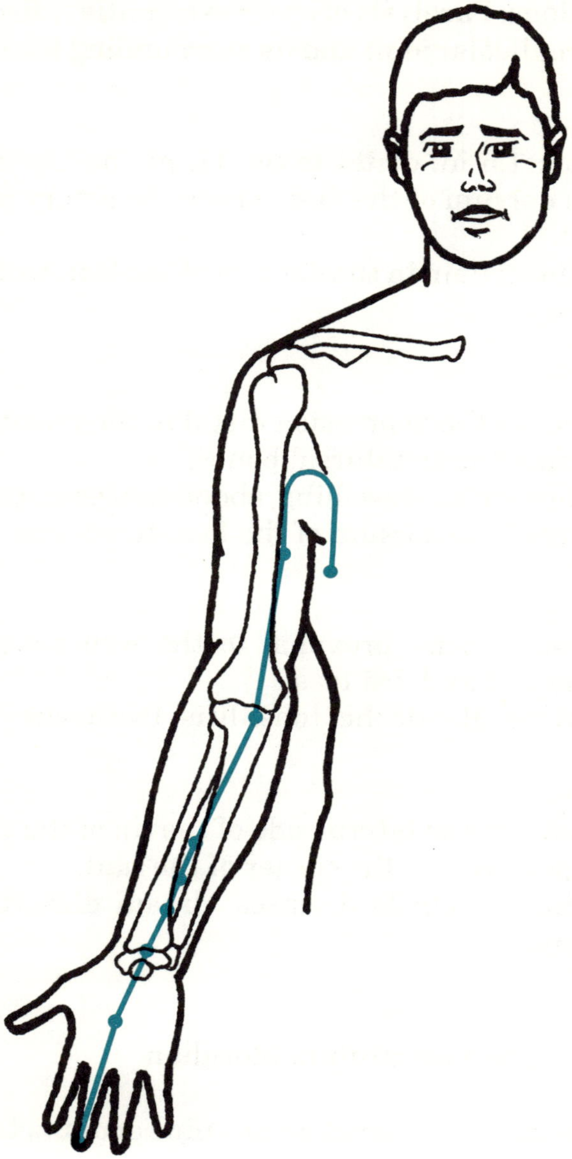

The Pericardium Meridian

Indications: Fullness in the chest, pain in the hypochrondiac region, tuberculosis of the lymph nodes.

2. P. 2 -

Location: 2 in. below the anterior end of the axillary fold, between the two heads of the biceps brachii muscle.

Indications: Pain in the chest and hypochrondriac region, cough, pain in the back and medial aspect of the arm.

3. P. 3 -

Location: In the middle of the transverse cubital crease, at the ulnar side of the tendon of the biceps brachii muscle.

Indications: Fever, palpitation, angina pectoris.

4. P. 4 -

Location: 5 in. above the transverse crease of the wrist, between the tendons of the palmaris longus and the flexor carpi radialis.

Indications: Tachycardia, angina pectoris, pleuritis, mastitis, neurasthenia.

5. P. 5 -

Location: 3 in. above the transverse crease of the wrist, between the tendons of the palmaris longus and the flexor carpi radialis.

Indications: Palpitation, angina pectoris, malaria, epilepsy.

6. P. 6 -

Location: 1 in. below P. 5, 2 in. above the wrist.

Indications: Vomiting, insomnia, palpitation, angina pectoris, hysteria, epilepsy, pain in the chest and costal region, hiccough.

7. P. 7 -

Location: At the midpoint of the transverse crease between the tendons of palmaris longus and flexor carpi radialis.

Indications: Insomnia, palpitation, epilepsy, disorders of the wrist joint and its surrounding soft tissue.

8. P. 8 -

Location: In the middle of the palm, between the middle and ring fingers, adjacent to the 3rd metacarpal bone.

Indication: Stomatitis, epilepsy, chronic skin infection of the hand, hiccough.

9. P. 9 -

Location: At the midpoint of the tip of the middle finger.

Indications: Coma, heat stroke, febrile diseases.

12

The Spleen Meridian

The Spleen meridian contains 21 acupuncture points. The points are located as follows:

1. Sp. 1 -
   Location: On the medial side of the great toe, 0.1 in. posterior to the corner of the nail.
   Indications: Abdominal distention, insomnia, irregular menstruation.

2. Sp. 2 -
   Location: On the medial side of the great toe, anterior and inferior to the 1st metatarso-phalangeal joint.
   Indications: Abdominal distention, abdominal pain, high fever.

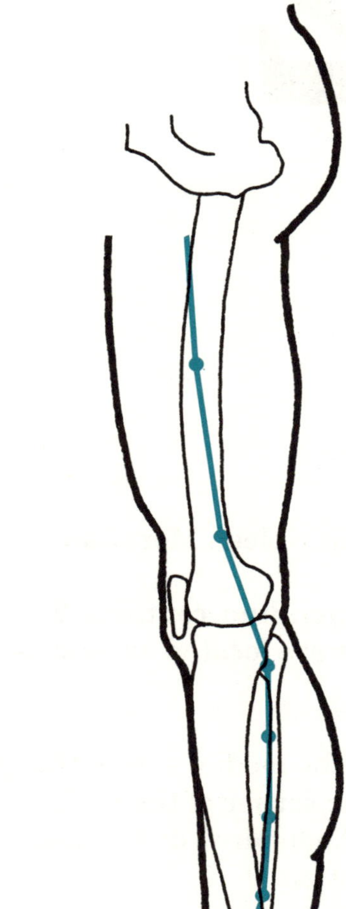

The Spleen Meridian

3. Sp. 3 -

Location: At the medial aspect of the foot, posterior and inferior to the head of the 1st metatarsal bone.

Indications: Abdominal distention, vomiting and diarrhea, constipation.

4. Sp. 4 -

Location: On the medial aspect of the foot, in a depression at the anterior and inferior border of the 1st metatarsal bone.

Indications: diarrhea, vomiting, dyspepsia.

5. Sp.5 -

Location: Draw a straight line along the anterior and inferior border of the medial malleolus respectively. The point is where the two lines cross.

Indications: Gastritis, enteritis, dyspepsia, pain in the ankle joint.

6. Sp. 6 -

Location: 3 in. above the tip of the medial malleolus just posterior to the tibial border.

Indications: Abdominal distention, irregular menstruation, impotence, orchitis, enuresis, frequency of urination, retention of urine, neurasthenia.

7. Sp. 7 -

Location: 3 in. in the depression above Sp. 6, at the posterior border of the tibia.

Indications: Abdominal distention, numbness of the leg.

8. Sp. 8 -

Location: 3 in. below Sp. 9 at the posterior border of the tibia.

Indications: Lumbago, edema, enuresis, nocturnal emission, menorrhagia.

9. Sp. 9 -
Location: In the depression on the lower border of the medial condyle of the tibia, on a level with the tuberosity of the tibia.
Indications: Abdominal distention, edema, dysuria, enuresis, inflammation of the inguinal lymph nodes.

10. Sp. 10 -
Location: 2 in. above the superior border of the patella, at the middle of the bulge of the vastus medialis muscle.
Indications: Irregular menstruation, functional uterine bleeding, urticaria.

11. Sp. 11 -
Location: 6 in. above Sp. 10, medial to the sartorius muscle.
Indications: Dysuria, eneuresis, inflammation of the inguinal lymph nodes.

12. Sp. 12 -
Location: On the lateral side of the femoral artery, 3.5 in. lateral to the midpoint of the superior border of the symphysis pubis.
Indications: Orchitis, endometritis, hernia.

13. Sp. 13 -
Location: 0.7 in. above Sp. 12, 4 in. lateral to abdominal midline.
Indications: Abdominal pain, hernia, appendicitis, constipation.

14. Sp. 14 -

Location: 1.3 in. below Spleen 15, 4 in. lateral to abdominal midline.

Indications: Peri-umbilical pain, hernia, diarrhea.

15. Sp. 15 -

Location: 4 in. lateral to the umbilicus, directly below the nipple, on the lateral side of the rectus abdominal muscle.

Indications: Abdominal pain, dyspepsia, intestinal paralysis, diarrhea.

16. Sp. 16 -

Location: 3 in. above Sp. 15.

Indications: Abdominal pain, constipation, dysentery.

17. Sp. 17 -

Location: In the 5th intercostal space, 6 in. lateral to the abdominal midline.

Indications: Pain and distention of chest and hyperchondriac region.

18. Sp. 18 -

Location: In the 4th intercostal space, 6 in. lateral to the abdominal midline.

Indications: Cough, mastitis, deficient lactation.

19. Sp. 19 -

Location: In the 3rd intercostal space, 6 in. lateral to the abdominal midline.

Indications: Pain and distention in the chest, costal and hyperchrondiac region.

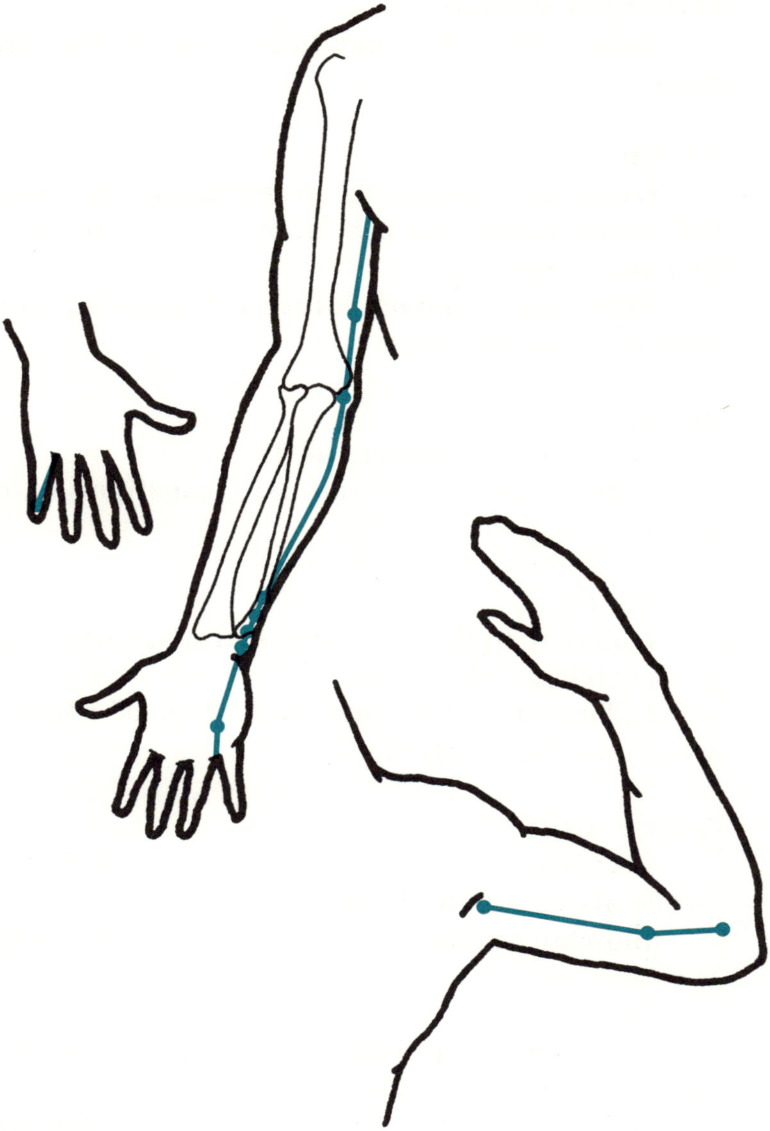

The Heart Meridian

20. Sp. 20 -

Location: In the 2nd interspace, 6 in. lateral to the abdominal midline.

Indications: Pain and distention of the chest, costal and hypochondriac region, cough.

21. Sp. 21 -

Location: On the midaxillary line, in the 6th costal interspace.

Indications: Pain in the chest, costal and hyperchrondriac region, dyspnea, general aching, weakness of the limbs.

The Heart Meridian

The Heart meridian contains 9 acupuncture points. They are as follows:

1. H. 1 -

Location: At the center of the axilla, on the medial side of the axillary artery.

Indications: Pain in the arm, paralysis of upper extremities, pain in the cardiac region, disorder of the shoulder joint and its surrounding tissue.

2. H. 2 -

Location: 3 in. above the elbow, in the groove medial to the biceps brachii muscle.

Indications: Pain in the costal and hyperchrondiac region, shoulder and arm.

3. H. 3 -

Location: Between the medial end of the transverse cubital crease and the medial epicondyle of the humerus when the elbow is bent.

Indications: Numbness of the hand and arm, tremor of the forearm, angina pectoris, disorders of the cubital joint and its surrounding soft tissue.

4. H. 4 -

Location: On the ulnar aspect proximal to the wrist, on the radial side of the tendon of flexor carpi ulnaris muscle, 1.5 in. above H. 7.

Indications: Angina Pectoris, ulnar neuralgia, pain in joints.

5. H. 5 -

Location: On the ulnar side of the wrist, on the radial side of the flexor carpi ulnaris muscle, 1 in. above H. 7.

Indications: Sudden hoarseness of voice, palpitation, pain in wrist and arm, stiffness of the tongue.

6. H. 6 -

Location: On the ulnar side of the wrist, on the radial side of the flexor carpi ulnaris muscle, 0.5 in. above H. 7.

Indications: Neurasthenia, angina pectoris, palpitation, night sweating.

7. H. 7 -

Location: On the ulnar side of the wrist, on the posterior border of the pisiform bone, in the depression on the radial side of the tendon of flexor carpi ulnaris muscle.

Indications: Insomnia, anxiety, palpitation, hysteria.

8. H. 8 -

Location: In the palmar surface, between the 4th and 5th metacarpal bones, just between the ring finger and small finger when making a fist.

Indications: Palpitation, pruritis vulvae, enuresis, elevated temperature on the palm of the hand.

9. H. 9 -

Location: On the radial side of the tip of the small finger, about 0.1 in. posterior to the corner of nail.

Indications: Palpitation, apoplexy, coma.

The Small Intestine Meridian

The Small Intestine meridian contains 19 acupuncture points. They are as follows:

1. S.I. 1 -

Location: At the ulnar side of the small finger, about 0.1 in. posterior to the corner of the nail.

Indications: Headache, eye diseases, mastitis.

2. S.I. 2 -

Location: In the depression anterior to the ulnar side of the 5th metacarpo-phalangeal joint.

Indications: Pain in the arm, numbness of the fingers, eye diseases, febrile diseases, tinnitus.

3. S.I. 3 -

Location: At the end of the transverse crease proximal to the 5th metacarpo-phalangeal joint when hand is half-clenched.

Indications: Stiffness or rigidity of the neck, tinnitus, occipital headache, lumbago, paralysis of the upper extremities, night sweating.

4. S.I. 4 -

Location: At the ulnar side of the border of the

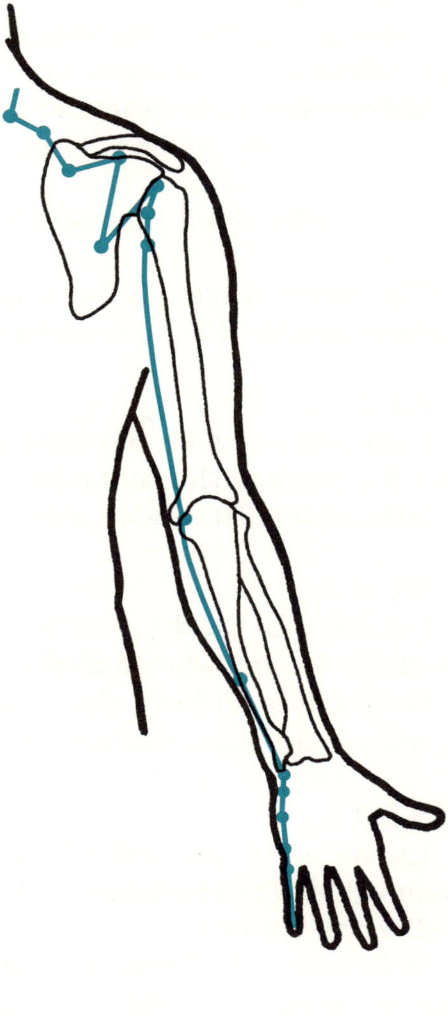

The Small Intestine Meridian

palm in the depression between the base of the 5th metacarpal bone and the trigonal bone.

Indications: Arthritis of the elbow, wrist and finger joints, headache, tinnitus, vomiting, cholescystitis.

5. S.I. 5 -

Location: At the ulnar side of the wrist in the depression between the styloid process of the ulna and the pisiform bone.

Indications: Swelling of the neck and submaxillary region, pain in the lateral aspect of the arm and wrist.

6. S.I. 6 -

Location: Flex elbow with arm placed on the chest, the point is on the bony cleft on the radial aspect of the styloid process of the ulna.

Indications: Pain in the wrist and back, paralysis of the upper extremities.

7. S.I. 7 -

Location: 5 in. proximal to the wrist, on a line connecting S.I. 5 with S.I. 8.

Indications: Rigidity or stiffness of the neck, pain in the elbow, arm and fingers.

8. S.I. 8 -

Location: In the posterior aspect of the cubital joint, in a depression between the olecranon of the ulna and the tip of the medial epicondyle of the humerus.

Indications: Pain in the small finger, elbow joint, shoulder and back.

9. S.I. 9 -

Location: With arm at the side, the point is 1 in. superior to the posterior axillary fold.

Indications: Pain in arm, paralysis of the upper extremities, disorders of the shoulder joint and its surrounding soft tissue.

10. S.I. 10 -

Location: With arm at the side, it is directly above the posterior axillary fold, on the lower border of the scapular spine.

Indications: Pain and weakness of shoulder and arm.

11. S.I. 11 -

Location: It is in the center of the infrascapular fossa forming a bilateral triangle with S.I. 10 and S.I. 9.

Indications: Pain in the shoulder and postero-lateral aspect of the elbow and arm.

12. S.I. 12 -

Location: In the center of the suprascapular fossa, directly above S.I. 11.

Indications: Pain in the shoulder joint, numbness and aching of upper extremities.

13. S.I. 13 -

Location: On the medial end of the suprascapular fossa, midway between S.I. 10 and the spinous process of the 2nd throacic vertebra.

Indications: Pain and contracture of the shoulder joint.

14. S.I. 14 -

Location: 3 in. lateral to the lower border of the

spinous process of the 1st thoracic vertebra, on a vertical line drawn from the vertebral border of the scapula.

Indications: Aching of scapular joint, stiffness and pain of neck.

15. S.I. 15 -

Location: 2 in. lateral to the lower border of the spinous process of the 7th cervical vertebra.

Indications: Pain in the shoulder and back, stiffness and pain in neck, bronchitis, asthma.

16. S.I. 16 -

Location: On the posterior border of the sterno-cleido-mastoid muscle, 0.5 in. posterior to L.I. 16.

Indications: Sore throat, rigidity and stiffness of the neck.

17. S.I. 17 -

Location: Posterior to the angle of the jaw on the anterior border of the sterno-cleido-mastoid muscle.

Indications: Tonsillitis, sore throat, aphasia.

18. S.I. 18 -

Location: Directly below the outer canthus, in the depression below the lower border of the zygomatic bone.

Indications: Facial paralysis, toothache, trigeminal neuralgia.

19. S.I. 19 -

Location: In the depression between the tragus and mandibular joint when the mouth is slightly opened.

Indications: Tinnitus, deafness, earache.

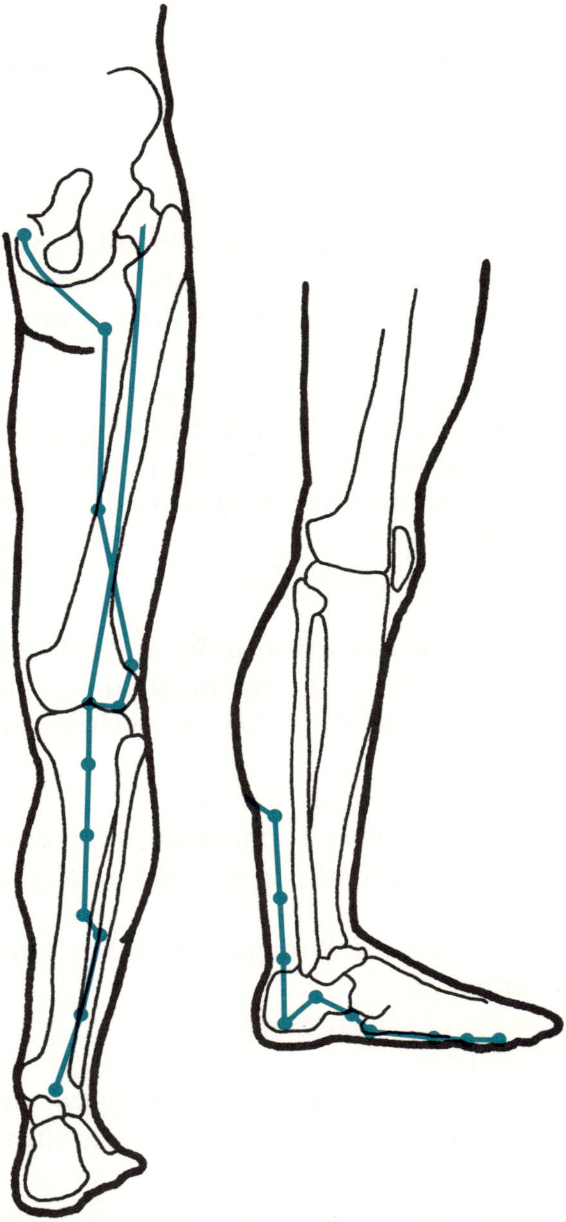

The Urinary Bladder Meridian

The Urinary Bladder Meridian

The Urinary Bladder meridian contains 67 acupuncture points. They are as follows:

1. U.B. 1 -

    Location: 0.1 in. lateral and superior to the inner canthus, near the medial orbital border.

    Indications: Eye diseases, facial paralysis.

2. U.B. 2 -

    Location: In the depression proximal to the medial end of the eyebrow, directly above the inner canthus.

    Indications: Headache, eye diseases, facial paralysis.

3. U.B. 3 -

    Location: Directly above U.B. 2, 0.5 in. inside the hairline.

    Indications: Headache, lacrimation, redness and swelling of the eye, blurring of vision.

4. U.B. 4 -

    Location: 1.5 in. lateral to U.B. 3, inside the hairline.

    Indications: Frontal headache, nasal obstruction, epistaxis.

5. U.B. 5 -

    Location: 0.5 in. above U.B. 4.

    Indications: Headache, epilepsy.

6. U.B. 6 -

    Location: 1.5 in. posterior to U.B. 5.

    Indications: Headache, dizziness, common cold.

7. U.B. 7 -

Location: 1.5 in. posterior to U.B. 6.

Indications: Vertical headache, sinusitis, rhinitis.

8. U.B. 8 -

Location: 1.5 in. posterior to U.B. 7.

Indications: Rhinitis, epistaxis, vertical headache, chronic bronchitis.

9. U.B. 9 -

Location: On the lateral side of the superior border of the external occipital protuberance.

Indications: Dizziness, vertical headache, myopia.

10. U.B. 10 -

Location: 1.3 in. lateral to the trapezius muscle below U.B. 9.

Indications: Occipital headache, stiffness and rigidity of the neck, insomnia, pharyngitis.

11. U.B. 11 -

Location: 1.5 in. lateral to the lower border of the spinous process of the 1st thoracic vertebra.

Indications: cough, fever, aching of the shoulder joint.

12. U.B. 12 -

Location: 1.5 in. lateral to the lower border of the 2nd thoracic vertebra.

Indications: common cold, bronchitis, urticaria.

13. U.B. 13 -

Location: 1.5 in. lateral to the lower border of the 3rd thoracic vertebra.

Indications: Cough, dyspnea, pulmonary tuberculosis, pneumonia, lesion of the soft tissue of the back of the neck.

14. U.B. 14 -
Location: 1.5 in. lateral to the lower border of the spinous process of the 4th thoracic vertebra.
Indications: Neurasthenia, fullness of the chest, vertical headache, pericarditis, hiccough.

15. U.B. 15 -
Location: 1.5 in. lateral to the lower border of the spinous process of the 5th thoracic vertebra.
Indications: Neurasthenia, cardiac diseases, epilepsy, schizophrenia.

16. U.B. 16 -
Location: 1.5 in. lateral to the lower border of the spinous process of the 6th thoracic vertebra.
Indications: Endocarditis, abdominal pain, hiccough, falling out of hair, pruritis of the skin.

17. U.B. 17 -
Location: 1.5 in. lateral to the lower border of the spinous process of the 7th thoracic vertebra.
Indications: Chronic hemorrhagic diseases, anemia, hiccough, nausea and vomiting, pain in the back, paralysis of the diaphragm muscle, pruritis.

18. U.B. 18 -
Location: 1.5 in. lateral to the lower border of the spinous process of the 9th thoracic vertebra.
Indications: Infectious hepatitis, hepatomegaly, cholecystitis, back pain, chronic eye diseases.

19. U.B. 19 -

Location: 1.5 in. lateral to the lower border of the spinous process of the 10th thoracic vertebra.

Indications: Infectious hepatitis, cholecystitis, back pain.

20. U.B. 20 -

Location: 1.5 in. lateral to the lower border of the spinous process of the 11th thoracic vertebra.

Indications: Gastric pain, gastric ulcer, chronic diarrhea, hepatitis, malaria, chronic hemorrhagic diseases, edema.

21. U.B. 21 -

Location: 1.5 in. lateral to the lower border of the spinous process of the 12th thoracic vertebra.

Indications: Gastric ulcer, nausea and vomiting, gastroptosis, chronic diarrhea.

22. U.B. 22 -

Location: 1.5 in. lateral to the lower border of the spinous process of the 1st lumbar vertebra.

Indications: Enteritis, nephritis, lumbago, enuresis.

23. U.B. 23 -

Location: 1.5 in. lateral to the lower border of the 2nd lumbar vertebra.

Indications: Nephritis, enuresis, impotence, irregular menstruation, chronic diarrhea, lumbago.

24. U.B. 24 -

Location: 1.5 in. lateral to the lower border of the 3rd lumbar vertebra.

Indications: lumbago, hemorrhoids.

25. U.B. 25 -

Location: 1.5 in. lateral to the lower border of the spinous process of 4th lumbar vertebra.

Indications: Lumbago, sprain of the lumbar region, diarrhea, constipation, dysentery, sciatica, paralysis of the lower extremities.

26. U.B. 26 -

Location: 1.5 in. lateral to the lower border of the 5th lumbar vertebra.

Indications: Lumbago, diarrhea, urogenital diseases.

27. U.B. 27 -

Location: 1.5 in. lateral to the midline of the back, level to the 1st posterior sacral foramen, in the depression between the medial border of the posterior superior iliac spine and the sacrum.

Indications: Lumbago, pain in the lumbosacral region, disorder of the sacroiliac joint, enteritis, hematuria.

28. U.B. 28 -

Location: Level with the 2nd sacral foramen, in the depression between the lower medial border of the posterior superior iliac spine and the sacrum.

Indications: Retention of urine, enuresis, pain in the lumbo-sacral region.

29. U.B. 29 -

Location: At the level of the 3rd posterior sacral foramen, 1.5 in. lateral to the midline of the back.

Indications: Enteritis, pain in the lumbo-sacral region, sciatica.

30. U.B. 30 -

Location: At the level of the 4th posterior sacral foramen, 1.5 in. lateral to the midline of the back.

Indications: Sciatica, sacral neuralgia, endometritis, hernia.

31. U.B. 31 -

Location: In the 1st posterior sacral foramen, about 1.5 in. from the midline of the back.

Indications: Orchitis, irregular menstruation, urogenital diseases, lumbago, sciatica, hemorrhoids, neurasthenia.

32. U.B. 32 -

Location: In the 2nd posterior sacral foramen, about midway between the midline of the back and the inferior aspect of the posterior superior iliac spine.

Indications: Orchitis, irregular menstruation, urogenital diseases, lumbago, sciatica, hemorrhoids, neurasthenia.

33. U.B. 33 -

Location: In the 3rd posterior sacral foramen, about midway between the midline of the back and U.B. 29.

Indications: Same as U.B. 31.

34. U. B. 34 -

Locations: In the 4th posterior sacral foramen, about midway between the midline of the back and U.B. 30.

Indications: Same as U.B. 31.

NOTE: In locating the above 4 points (U.B. 31, 32, 33, 34) place the tip of the index finger midway between U.B. 27 and mid-point of the spinal column with the little finger on the sacral prominence, place the middle and ring finger equidistance to each other. The spot of contact of the index finger is the upper sacral foramen, the spot under the tip of the middle finger is the 2nd sacral foramen and that under the tip of the ring finger is the 3rd sacral foramen, while the 4th sacral foramen is under the tip of the little finger.

35. U.B. 35 -

Location: Lateral to the lower end of the coccyx, 0.5 in. lateral to the midline.

Indications: Back pain during menstruation, impotence, diarrhea, hemorrhoids.

36. U.B. 36 -

Location: Midpoint to the gluteal fold.

Indications: Sciatica, paralysis of the lower extremities, hemorrhoids.

37. U.B. 37 -

Location: On a line connecting the midpoints of the gluteal transverse crease and the popliteal transverse crease, 6 in. below the former.

Indications: Sciatica, back pain, paralysis of the lower extremities.

38. U.B. 38 -

Location: 1 in. above U.B. 39.

Indications: Cystitis, constipation, paralysis of the lower aspect of lower extremities.

39. U.B. 39 -

Location: On the lateral end of the popliteal crease, lateral to U.B. 40, on the medial side of the tendon of the biceps femoral muscle.

Indications: Spasm of the gastrocnemius muscle,

back pain.

40. U.B. 40 -

Location: Exact midpoint of the popliteal transverse crease.

Indications: Sciatica, back pain, paralysis of the lower extremities, disorder of the femoral joint and surrounding soft tissue.

41. U.B. 41 -

Location: 3 in. lateral to the lower border of the spinous process of the 2nd thoracic vertebra.

Indications: Intercostal neuralgia, numbness of the elbow and arm.

42. U.B. 42 -

Location: 3 in. lateral to the lower border of the spinous process of the 3rd thoracic vertebra.

Indications: Bronchitis, asthma, pleuritis, vomiting, shoulder pain.

43. U.B. 43 -

Location: 3 in. lateral to the lower border of the spinous process of the 4th thoracic vertebra.

Indications: Bronchitis, pleuritis, general weakness.

44. U.B. 44 -

Location: 3 in. lateral to the lower border of the spinous process of the 5th thoracic vertebra.

Indications: Cardiac diseases, bronchitis, asthma, shoulder and back pain.

45. U.B. 45 -

Location: 3 in. lateral to the lower border of the spinous process of the 6th thoracic vertebra.

Indications: Pericarditis, intercostal neuralgia, hiccough, vomiting, dizziness and vertigo, asthma.

46. U.B. 46 -

Location: 3 in. lateral to the lower border of the spinous process of the 7th thoracic vertebra.

Indications: Intercostal neuralgia, vomiting, hiccough, pain in the spinal column.

47. U.B. 47 -

Location: 3 in. lateral to the lower border of the spinous process of the 9th thoracic vertebra.

Indications: Liver diseases, pleuritis, endocarditis, dyspepsia.

48. U.B. 48 -

Location: 3 in. lateral to the lower border of the spinous process of the 10th thoracic vertebra.

Indications: Diarrhea, abdominal pain, jaundice.

49. U.B. 49 -

Location: 3 in. lateral to the lower border of the spinous process of the 11th thoracic vertebra.

Indications: Back pain, abdominal distention, liver diseases, vomiting.

50. U.B. 50 -

Location: 3 in. lateral to the lower border of the spinous process of the 12th thoracic vertebra.

Indications: Vomiting, abdominal distention, constipation, pain in the spinal column.

51. U.B. 51 -

Location: 3 in. lateral to the lower border of the spinous process of the 1st lumbar vertebra.

Indications: Upper abdominal pain, constipation, mastitis, hepatomegaly, splenomegaly.

52. U.B. 52 -

Location: 3 in. lateral to the lower border of the spinous process of the 2nd lumbar vertebra.

Indications: Stiffness and pain in the back and lumbar region.

53. U.B. 53 -

Location: 3 in. lateral to the lower border of the 2nd posterior sacral vertebra.

Indications: Enteritis, abdominal distention, back pain, retention of urine.

54. U.B. 54 -

Location: 3 in. lateral to the lower border of the 4th posterior sacral veterbra.

Indications: Cystitis, hemorrhoids, sciatica, paralysis and numbness or pain of the lower extremities.

55. U.B. 55 -

Location: 2 in. directly below, U.B. 40 on a line connecting U.B. 40 with U.B. 57.

Indications: Lumbago and leg pain, paralysis of the lower extremities.

56. U.B. 56 -

Location: Midway between U.B. 55 and U.B. 57 in the center of the belly of the gastrocnemius muscle.

Indications: Leg pain, hemorrhoids, stiffness and pain in the back and lumbar region.

57. U.B. 57 -

Location: Midway between U.B. 40 and the heel, on the groove 8 in. below U.B. 40.

Indications: Sciatica, prolapse of the rectum, spasm of the gastrocnemius, pain in the sole, paralysis of the lower extremities.

58. U.B. 58 -

Location: 7 in. directly above U.B. 60, posterior to the external malleolus.

Indications: Lumbago, leg pain, nephritis, cystitis, weakness in legs.

59. U.B. 59 -

Location: 3 in. above U.B. 60, posterior to the external malleolus.

Indications: Headache, pain in the lumbo-sacral region, pain and swelling of the ankle region.

60. U.B. 60

Location: Between the posterior border of the external malleolus and the medial aspect of the tendo calcaneus, at the same level as the tip of the malleolus.

Indications: Paralysis of the lower extremity, lumbago, sciatica, disorder of the ankle joint and surrounding tissue.

61. U.B. 61 -

Location: 1.5 in. inferior to the external malleolus, directly below U.B. 60, posterior to the calcaneus.

Indications: Painful heel, weakness or paralysis of the lower extremities.

62. U.B. 62 -

Location: Directly below the tip of the external malleolus, and 0.5 in. lateral to its lower border.

Indications: Epilepsy, headache, dizziness and vertigo.

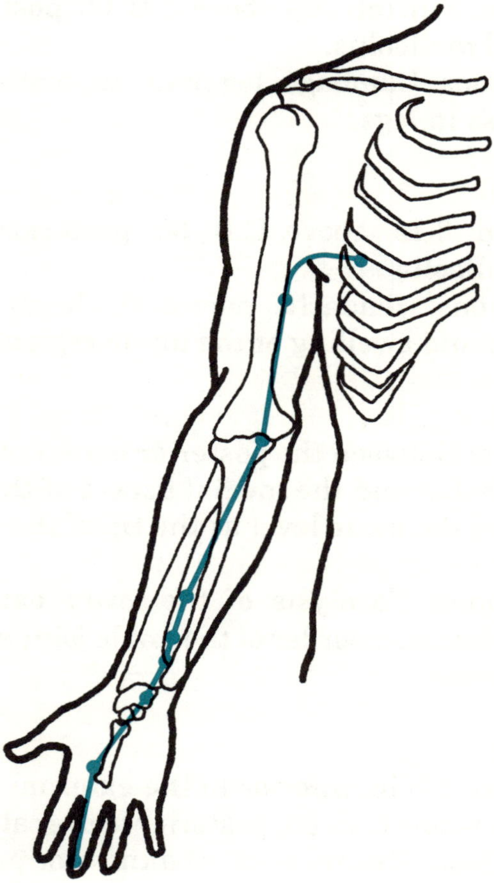

The Heart Constrictor Meridian

63. U.B. 63 -

Location: Anterior and inferior to U.B. 62, in the depression posterior to the tuberosity of the 5th metatarsal bone.

Indications: Pain around the ankle joint, lumbago, pain in the leg.

64. U.B. 64 -

Location: Below the tuberosity of the 5th metatarsal bone.

Indications: Headaches, dizziness and vertigo, lumbago and leg pain.

65. U.B. 65 -

Location: Posterior and inferior to the small head of the 5th metatarsal bone.

Indications: Headaches, pain, lumbago, leg pain.

66. U.B. 66 -

Location: In the depression anterior and inferior to the 5th metatarso-phalangeal joint.

Indications: Headache, dizziness, epistaxis.

67. U.B. 67 -

Location: On the lateral side of the tip of the small toe, about 0.1 in. posterior to the corner of the nail.

Indications: Malposition of the fetus, difficult labor.

The Heart Constrictor Meridian

The Heart Constrictor Meridian has 9 acupuncture points. They are as follows:

1. HC 1 -

Location: 1 in lateral to the nipple in the 4th intercostal space.

Indications: Fullness in the chest, pain in the hypochrondiac region, tuberculosis of the lymph nodes.

2. HC 2 -

Location: 2 in. below the end of the axillary fold, between the two heads of the biceps brachii muscle.

Indications: Pain in the chest and the hypochondriac region, cough, pain in the back and medial aspect of the arm.

3. HC 3 -

Location: In the middle of the transverse cubital crease, at the ulnar side of the tendon of the biceps muscle.

Indications: Fever, palpitation, angina pectoris.

4. HC 4 -

Location: 5 in. above the transverse crease of the wrist, between the tendons of the palmaris longus and the flexor carpi radialis muscles.

Indications: Tachycardia, angina pectoris, pleuritis, mastitis, neurasthenia.

5. HC 5 -

Location: 3 in. above the transverse crease of the wrist, between the tendons of the palmaris longus and flexor carpi radialis muscles.

Indications: Palpitation, angina pectoris, malaria, epilepsy, schizophrenia.

6. HC 6 -

Location: 1 in. below HC 5, 2 in. above the wrist.

Indications: Vomiting, insomnia, palpitation,

angina pectoris, hysteria, pain in chest and costal region, spasm of the diaphragm (hiccough).

7. HC 7 -

Location: At the midpoint of the transverse crease of the wrist between the tendons of the palmaris longus and flexor carpi radialis muscles.

Indications: Insomnia, palpitation, epilepsy, disorders of the wrist joint and its surrounding soft tissue.

8. HC 8 -

Location: In the middle of the palm, between the middle and the ring fingers, adjacent to the 3rd metacarpal bone.

Indications: Stomatitis, epilepsy, chronic skin infection of the hand, hiccough.

9. HC 9 -

Location: At the midpint of the tip of the middle finger.

Indications: Coma, heat stroke, febrile diseases.

The Tri-Heater Meridian

The Tri-Heater meridian contains 23 acupuncture points. They are as follows:

1. TH 1 -

Location: On the ulnar side of the ring finger, 0.1 in. posterior to the corner of the nail.

Indications: Headache, sore throat, febrile diseases.

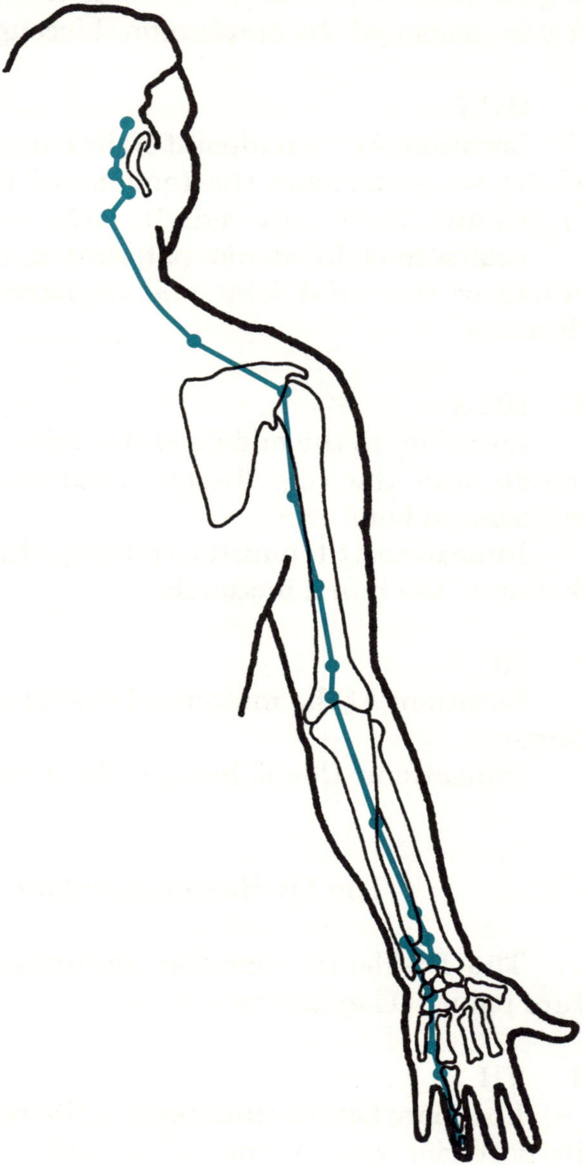

The Tri-Heater Meridian

2. TH 2 -

Location: 0.5 in. proximal to the margin of the web between the ring and the small fingers.

Indications: Headache, conjunctivitis, deafness, sore throat, pain in hand and arm.

3. TH 3 -

Location: On the dorsum of the hand between the 4th and 5th metacarpal bones, in a depression posterior to the metacarpophalangeal joint.

Indications: Deafness, tinnitus, headache, sore throat, and paralysis of the upper extremities or hands.

4. TH 4 -

Location: In a depression of the transverse crease of the dorsum of the wrist, between the extensor digitorum communis and the extensor digit quinti proprius.

Indications: Disorder of the wrist joint and its surrounding soft tissue.

5. TH 5 -

Location: 2 in. above the transverse crease of the dorsum of the wrist between the radius and the ulna.

Indications: Paralysis of the upper extremities, thoraco-costal pain, headache, deafness, tinnitus, stiff neck, common cold, fever.

6. TH 6 -

Location: 1 in. above TH 5, between the ulna and the radius.

Indications: Constipation, shoulder and back pain, thoraco-cos pain, sore throat, fever, paralysis of the upper extremities.

7. TH 7 -

Location: About 1 finger breadth lateral to TH 6, on the radial side of the ulna.

Indications: Deafness, pain in the upper extremities, epilepsy.

8. TH 8 -

Location: 1 in. above TH 6, between the radius and ulna.

Indications: Deafness, pain in the arm, aphasia.

9. TH 9 -

Location: 5 in. below the olecranon, between the radius and the ulna.

Indications: Deafness, toothache, pain in the forearm.

10. TH 10 -

Location: 1 in. posterior and superior to the olecranon, in the depression made by flexing the elbow.

Indications: Disorders of the elbow joint and its surrounding soft tissue.

11. TH 11 -

Location: 1 in. above TH 10. Flex elbow to locate this point.

Indications: Pain in the shoulder and arm.

12. TH 12 -

Location: Midway between TH 11 and TH 13.

Indications: Headache, pain in the arm.

13. TH 13 -

Location: 3 in. below TH 14 at the posterior border of the deltoid.

Indications: Pain in the shoulder and arm, pain and swelling of the scapular joint, eye diseases.

14. TH 14 -

Location: When the arm is raised horizontally, two depressions appear on the shoulder. The posterior one is the point.

Indications: Disorders of the shoulder joint and its surrounding soft tissue, Pain in arm and paralysis of the upper extremities.

15. TH 15 -

Location: Midway between the tip of the acromion, 1 in. inferior to GB 21.

Indications: Pain in shoulder and arm, motor impairment of arm, pain in neck.

16. TH 16 -

Location: Posterior and inferior to the mastoid process, on the posterior border of the sterno-cleido-mastoid muscle at the level of the angle of the mandible.

Indications: Deafness, rigidity of neck.

17. TH 17 -

Location: Posterior to the ear-lobe, in a depression between the angle of the mandible and mastoid process.

Indications: Deafness, tinnitus, otitis media, parotitis.

18. TH 18 -

Location: Posterior to the ear, in the center of the mastoid process, at the junction of the middle and lower third of the curve line connecting TH 20 with TH 17 along the helix.

Indications: Deafness, tinnitus, facial paralysis.

19. TH 19 -

Location: 1 in. above TH 18.

Indications: Tinnitus, vomiting, otitis media.

20. TH 20 -

Location: Fold ear forward; the point is within the hairline where the tip touches.

Indications: Redness and swelling of the ear, cloudiness of the cornea, toothache.

21. TH 21 -

Location: When mouth is open, the point is in the depression in front of the anterior notch of the auricle and slightly superior to the condyloid process of the mandible.

Indications: Deafness, tinnitus, otitis media.

22. TH 22 -

Location: On the hairline anterior and superior to TH 21, anterior to and level with the root of the auricle, posterior to the superficial temporal artery.

Indications: Tinnitus, headache, trismus, facial paralysis.

23. TH 23 -

Location: On the lateral border of the orbit at the lateral tip of the eyebrow.

Indications: Headache, eye diseases.

13

The Kidney Meridian

The Kidney meridian contains 27 acupuncture points. They are as follows:

1. K. 1 -

Location: In the depression at the junction of the anterior and middle third of the sole of the foot in a depression between the 2nd and 3rd metatarsophalangeal joint when the toes are plantar flexed.

Indication: Coma, shock, hysteria, epilepsy, nausea and vomiting, sore throat, vertical headache.

2. K. 2 -

Location: Anterior and inferior to the medial malleolus, in a depression at the anterior and inferior border of the navicular bone.

Indications: Cystitis, irregular menstruation,

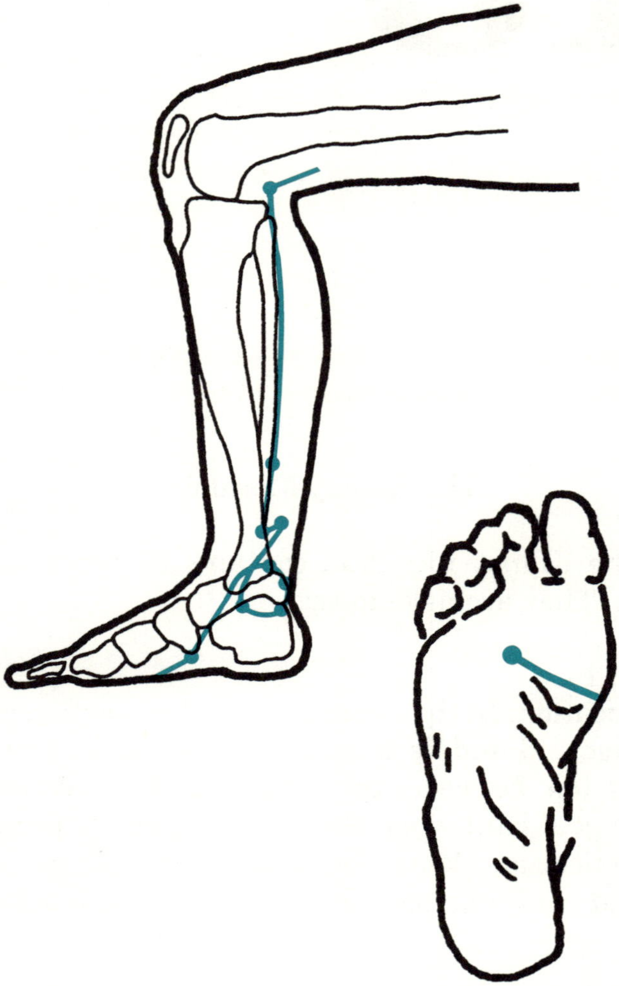

The Kidney Meridian

diabetes, sore throat.

3. K. 3 -

Location: Midway between the tip of the medial malleolus and the tendo calcaneus.

Indications: Nephritis, cystitis, enuresis, irregular menstruation, sore throat, toothache, paralysis of the lower extremities.

4. K. 4 -

Location: Inferior and anterior to the medial malleolus, in the depression medial to the attachment to the tendo calcaneus, 0.5 in. slightly posteriorly below K. 3.

Indications: Neurasthenia, hysteria, hemoptysis, asthma, constipation, painful heel.

5. K. 5 -

Location: 1 in. inferior to K. 3 in the depression anterior and superior to the medial side of the tubercle of the calcaneum.

Indications: Irregular menstruation, prolapse of the uterus, myopia.

6. K. 6 -

Location: In the depression 1 in. directly below the inferior border of the medial malleolus.

Indications: Irregular menstruation, prolapse of the uterus, tonsillitis, neurasthenia, epilepsy.

7. K. 7 -

Location: 2 in. above K. 3, on the anterior border of the tendo calcaneus.

Indications: Nephritis, orchitis, night sweating, diarrhea, lumbago, paralysis of the lower extremities.

8. K. 8 -

Location: 2 in. above K. 3, 0.5 in. anterior to K. 7, posterior to the medial border of the tibia.

Indications: Irregular menstruation, functional uterine bleeding, diarrhea, constipation, pain and swelling of the testis.

9. K. 9 -

Location: 5 in. above K. 3, about 1 in. posterior to the medial border of the tibia.

Indications: Spasm of the gastrocnemius muscle, epilepsy.

10. K. 10 -

Location: At the medial end of the popliteal transverse crease, between the tendons of the semitendosus and semimembranosus muscles.

Indications: Knee pain, lower abdominal pain, disorders of the genital system.

11. K. 11 -

Location: In the lower abdomen, on the superior border of the symphysis pubis.

Indications: Eneuresis, hernia, spermatorrhea, impotence.

12. K. 12 -

Location: 1 in. above K. 11.

Indications: Pain in the external genitalia, excessive leukorrhea.

13. K. 13 -

Location: 2 in. above K. 11.

Indications: Irregular menstruation, diarrhea.

14. K. 14 -

Location: 3 in. above K. 11.

Indications: Uterine Bleeding, postpartum abdominal pain, diarrhea.

15. K. 15 -

Location: 1 in. below umbilicus.

Indications: Irregular menstruation, lower abdominal pain, constipation.

16. K. 16 -

Location: 0.5 in. lateral to umbilicus.

Indications: Jaundice, hernia, constipation.

17. K. 17 -

Location: 2 in. above K. 16.

Indications: Abdominal pain, anorexia, hernia.

18. K. 18 -

Location: 3 in. above K. 16.

Indications: Hiccough, constipation, postpartum abdominal pain.

19. K. 19 -

Location: 4 in. above K. 16.

Indications: Abdominal pain, abdominal distention.

20. K. 20 -

Location: 5 in. above K. 16.

Indications: Vomiting, diarrhea, abdominal pain, abdominal distention.

21. K. 21 -

Location: 6 in. above K. 16.

Indications: Belching, vomiting, diarrhea.

22. K. 22 -
Location: In the 5th intercostal space, 7 in. above K. 16.
Indications: Intercostal neuralgia, pleurisy, bronchitis.

23. K. 23 -
Location: In the 4th intercostal space, directly above K. 22.
Indications: Intercostal neuralgia, pleurisy, bronchitis, mastitis.

24. K. 24 -
Location: In the 3rd intercostal interspace, above K. 23.
Indications: Pain in the chest and costal region, cough, vomiting, mastitis.

25. K. 25 -
Location: In the 2nd intercostal interspace, midway between the sternal and mammilary lines.
Indications: cough, vomiting, intercostal neuralgia.

26. K. 26 -
Location: In the 1st intercostal space, midway between the sternal and mammilary lines.
Indication: cough, chest pain, vomiting.

27. K. 27 -
Location: In the depression between the 1st rib and the lower border of the clavicle.
Indications: Chest pain, cough, asthma, vomiting.

The Gall Bladder Meridian

The Gall Bladder Meridian contains 44 acupuncture points. They are as follows:

1. G.B. 1 -

Location: 0.5 in. lateral to the outer canthus.

Indications: Eye diseases, headache, facial paralysis.

2. G.B. 2 -

Location: Posterior and anterior to the tragus, anterior to the tragus notch. There is a depression when the mouth is opened.

Indications: Deafness, tinnitus, otitis media, facial paralysis, arthritis of the mandibular joint.

3. G.B. 3 -

Location: In front of the ear, on the upper border of the zygomatic arch, directly above St. 7.

Indications: Facial paralysis. tinnitus, deafness, toothache.

4. G.B. 4 -

Location: 1 in. below St. 8 on the hairline of the temporal region. There is a slight movement during chewing.

Indications: Migraine, dizziness, tinnitus, rhinitis, facial paralysis.

5. G.B. 5 -

Location: In a line connecting G.B. 4 and G.B. 7, at the junction of anterior and midle third of the line.

Indications: Migraine, neurasthenia, toothache.

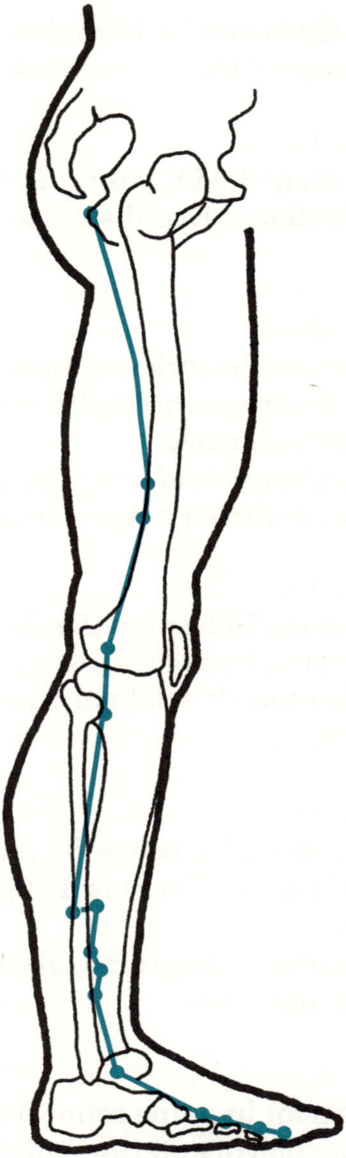

The Gall Bladder Meridian

6. G.B. 6 -

Location: In a line connecting G.B. 4 and G.B. 7, at the junction of the inferior and middle third of the line.

Indications: Migraine, neurasthenia, facial swelling, toothache.

7. G.B. 7 -

Location: At the crossing point of the horizontal line of the auricle and the line that projects from the anterior auricle.

Indications: Pain and swelling of the cheek and submaxillary region, difficulty in opening the mouth, headache, stiff neck.

8. G.B. 8 -

Location: Fold the ear over, the point is directly above the auricular apex, 1.5 in. within the hairline.

Indication: Migraine, dizziness and vertigo.

9. G.B. 9 -

Location: 0.5 in. posterior to G.B. 8, superior and posterior to the auricle, 2 in. inside the hair line.

Indications: Headache, swelling and pain of the gum, epilepsy.

10. G.B. 10 -

Location: About 1 in. inferior to G.B. 9, at the upper border of the root of the auricle, 1 in. beyond the hairline.

Indication: Tinnitus, deafness, toothache, tonsillitis.

11. G.B. 11 -

Location: Midpoint of the line connecting G.B. 10 and G.B. 12.

Indications: Vertical headache.

12. G.B. 12 -
Location: In the depression, posterior and inferior to the mastoid process. Ask the patient to bend his neck to locate the point.
Indications: Tinnitus, toothache, swelling of the cheek, facial paralysis.

13. G.B. 13 -
Location: 0.5 in. inside the hairline, directly above the outer canthus.
Indications: epilepsy, stiff neck.

14. G.B. 14 -
Location: 1 in. above the midpoint of the eyebrow.
Indications: Frontal headache, night blindness, glaucoma.

15. G.B. 15 -
Location: With the patient looking straight ahead, it is 0.5 in. inside the hairline, directly above the pupil.
Indications: Nasal obstruction, eye diseases.

16. G.B. 16 -
Location: 1 in. above G.B. 15.
Indications: eye diseases, facial swelling.

17. G.B. 17 -
Location: 1 in. posterior to G.B. 16.
Indications: Headache, toothache.

18. G.B. 18 -
Location: 1.5 in. posterior to G.B. 17.
Indications: Headache, nasal obstruction, epis-

taxis.

19. G.B. 19 -

Location: 1.5 in. above G.B.20, on the lateral side of the occipital protuberance.

Indications: Headache, stiff neck, epistaxis, asthma.

20. G.B. 20 -

Location: In a depression between the sternocleidomastoid muscle and the upper portion of the trapezius muscle. Specifically, between the depression directly inferior to the occipital protuberance and the mastoid.

Indications: Common cold, headache, dizziness and vertigo, stiffness of the neck, hypertension, tinnitus.

21. G.B. 21 -

Location: At the highest point of the shoulder at the acromion.

Indications: Pain in the shoulder and back, rigidity and stiffness of the neck, motor impairment of the upper extremities, mastitis, hyperthyroidism, functional uterine bleeding.

22. G.B. 22 -

Location: 3 in. below the anterior axillary fold, on the axillary line in the 4th intercostal space when the arm is raised.

Indications: Pleuritis, intercostal neuralgia, inflammation of the axillary lymph nodes.

23. G.B. 23 -

Location: 1 in. anterior to G.B. 22, in the 4th intercostal space.

Indications: Vomiting, gastric acidity, salivation, asthma.

24. G.B. 24 -

Location: One rib directly below Liv. 14, in the 7th intercostal space.

Indications: Hiccough, hepatitis, cholecystitis.

25. G.B. 25 -

Location: On the lateral side of the abdomen, at the lower border of the free end of the 12th rib.

Indications: Costal pain, abdominal distention.

26. G.B. 26 -

Location: Midway between the free ends of the 11th and 12th ribs, level with the umbilicus.

Indications: Endometritis, cystitis, lumbago, costal and back pain.

27. G.B. 27 -

Location: 3 in. anterior and inferior to G.B. 26, in front of the anterior superior iliac spine.

Indications: Pain in the lower abdomen, lumbago, endometritis, orchitis.

28. G.B. 28 -

Location: Anterior and inferior to the anterior superior iliac spine, 0.5 in. anterior and inferior to G.B. 27.

Indications: Endometritis, pain in lower abdomen, chronic constipation.

29. G.B. 29 -

Location: Midway between the anterior superior iliac spine and the highest point of the greater trochanter of the femur. Locate the point with the patient in the recumbent position.

Indications: Disorders of the hip joint and its surrounding soft tissue, pain in the lower extremities.

30. G.B. 30 -

Location: At the junction of the middle and lateral third of the distance between the highest point of the greater trochanter of the femur and the hiatus of the sacrum. Locate this point with the patient in lateral recumbent position with the thigh flexed.

Indications: Sciatica, paralysis of the lower extremities, disorders of the hip joint and its surrounding soft tissue.

31. G.B 31 -

Location: At the lateral side of the thigh, 7 in. above the transverse popliteal crease between the vastus lateralis muscle and the biceps femoris muscle. With the patient standing erect, hands close to thighs, the point is at the tip of the middle finger.

Indications: Paralysis of the lower extremities, pain in the lumbar region and legs, neurodermitis of the lateral aspect of the thigh.

32. G.B. 32 -

Location: On the lateral aspect of the thigh, 2 in. below G.B. 31.

Indications: Hemiplegia, sciatica.

33. G.B. 33 -

Location: In the depression superior to the lateral epicondyle of the femur, 3 in. above G.B. 34.

Indications: Pain in the knee joint.

34. G.B. 34 -

Location: In the depression anterior and inferior

to the small head of the fibula.

Indications: Hemiplegia, diseases of the gall bladder, lumbago and leg pain, dizziness and vertigo.

35. G.B. 35 -

Location: 7 in. above the tip of the external malleolus, in the anterior border of the fibula, on a line connecting the tip of the external malleolus with G.B. 34.

Indications: Pain in the lateral aspect of the leg, sciatica, asthma.

36. G.B. 36 -

Location: Level and 1 in. posterior to G.B. 35, and posterior to the border of the fibula.

Indications: Pain in the lateral aspect of the leg, spasm of the gastrocnemius muscle.

37. G.B. 37 -

Location: 5 in. above the tip of the external malleolus, close to the anterior border of the fibula.

Indications: Eye diseases, pain in the lower extremities.

38. G.B. 38 -

Location: 4 in. above the tip of the external malleolus, on the anterior border of the fibula.

Indications: Lumbago, arthritis of the knee joint, general malaise.

39. G.B. 39 -

Location: 3 in. above the external malleolus, between the posterior border of the fibula and the tendons of the peroneus longus and brevis muscle.

Indications: Paralysis of the lower extremities, stiffness and rigidity of the neck, disorders of the ankle joint and surrounding soft tissue.

40. G.B. 40 -

Location: Anterior and inferior to the external malleolus, in the depression on the lateral side of the extensor digitorum longus muscle.

Indications: Pain in the lower extremities, pain in the ankle joint.

41. G.B. 41 -

Location: In the depression anterior to the junction of the 4th and 5th metarsal bones.

Indications: Pain in foot, mastitis, tinnitus.

42. G.B. 42 -

Location: On the cleft between the 4th and 5th metarsal bones, 0.5 in. anterior to G,B. 41.

Indications: Tinnitus, pain in the axilla, mastitis.

43. G.B. 43 -

Location: On a cleft between the 4th and 5th metatarsal bones, 0.5 in. proximal to the margin of the web.

Indications: Deafness, headache, dizziness, chest pain, intercostal neuralgia.

44. G.B. 44 -

Location: On the lateral side of the tip of the 4th toe, 0.1 in. posterior to the corner of the nail.

Indications: Pleuritis, asthma, headache, pharyngitis.

The Liver Meridian

The Liver meridian contains 14 acupuncture

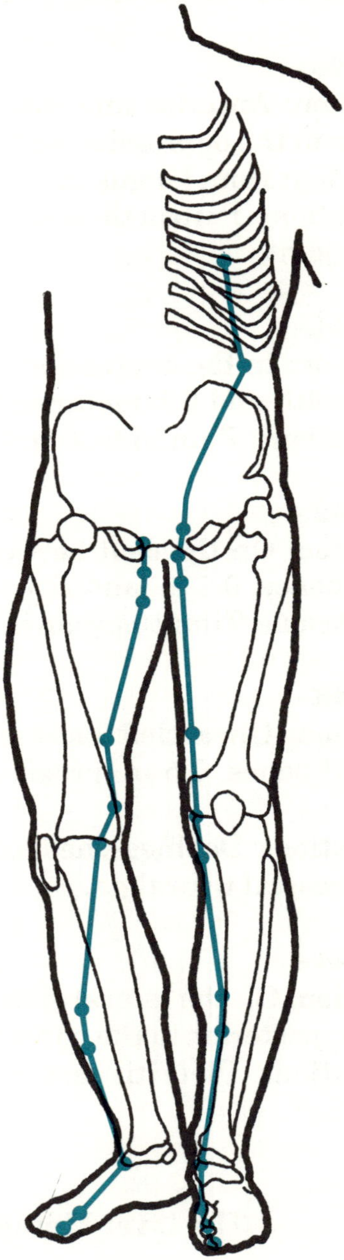

The Liver Meridian

points. They are as follows:

1. Liv. 1 -
   Location: On the lateral aspect of the dorsum of the terminal phalanx of the big toe, midway between the lateral corner of the nail and interphalangeal joint.
   Indications: Enuresis, menorrhagia, hernia.

2. Liv. 2 -
   Location: 0.5 in proximal to the margin of the web between the 1st and 2nd toes.
   Indications: Irregular menstruation, urethritis, enuresis, pain in the costal region, hypertension, epilepsy, insomnia, redness and swelling of the eye.

3. Liv. 3 -
   Location: Between the 1st and 2nd toe, 2 in. proximal to the margin of the web.
   Indications: Headache, dizziness, epilepsy, convulsions in children and infants, eye diseases, hernia. uterine bleeding, mastitis.

4. Liv. 4 -
   Location: 1 in. anterior to the medial malleolus, in the depression medial to the tendon of the tibialis anticus muscle.
   Indications: Pain in the lower abdomen, retention of urine, hernia, pain in the penis.

5. Liv. 5 -
   Location: 5 in. superior to the medial malleolus, on the posterior of the tibia.
   Indications: Inflammation of the pelvic organs, retention of urine, impotence.

6. Liv. 6 -

Location: 7 in. superior to the tip of the malleolus, on the posterior border of the tibia.

Indications: Irregular menstruation, hernia, pain in the joints of the lower extremities.

7. Liv. 7 -

Location: In the posterior and inferior aspect of the medial condyle of the tibia, 1 in. posterior to Sp. 9.

Indications: Pain in the knee joint.

8. Liv. 8 -

Location: At the medial end of the transverse crease of the knee joint, in a depression at the anterior border of the semimembranosus and semitendinosus muscles.

Indications: Infection in the urogenital system, impotence, hernia, disorders of the knee joint and its surrounding soft tissue.

9. Liv. 9 -

Location: 4 in. superior to the medial condyle of the femur, between the vastus medialis and sartorius muscles.

Indications: Lumbago, pain in the lower abdomen, enuresis, irregular menstruation.

10. Liv. 10 -

Location: 1 in. below Liv. 11 in the medial aspect of the thigh.

Indications: Distention in the lower abdomen, retention of urine, enuresis, eczema of the scrotum.

11. Liv. 11 -

Location: 1 in. inferior to the lateral aspect of the femoral artery in the inguinal groove. Locate the point with the patient in the supine position.

Indications: Femoral neuralgia, lumbago, pain in the leg, paralysis of lower extremities.

12. Liv. 12 -

Location: 2.5 in. lateral to and 1 in. inferior to the superior border of the symphysis pubis, at the lower portion of the inguinal groove.

Indications: Pain in the lower abdomen, prolapse of the uterus, pain in the lower abdomen, pain in the medial aspect of the thigh.

13. Liv. 13 -

Location: On the free end of the 11th rib.

Indications: Splenomegaly, diarrhea, abdominal distention, pain in the costal region.

14. Liv. 14 -

Location: On the mamillary line, directly below the nipple, in the intercostal space of the 6th and 7th ribs.

Indications: Pleuritis, hepatitis, chest pain, pain in the hypochrondriac region.

The Governing Vessel Meridian

The Governing Vessel meridian has 28 acupuncture points. They are as follows:

1. Gv. 1 -

Location: Midway between the tip of the coccyx and the anus, located with the patient in the prone or knee-chest position.

Indications: Hemorrhoids, prolapse of the rectum, diarrhea.

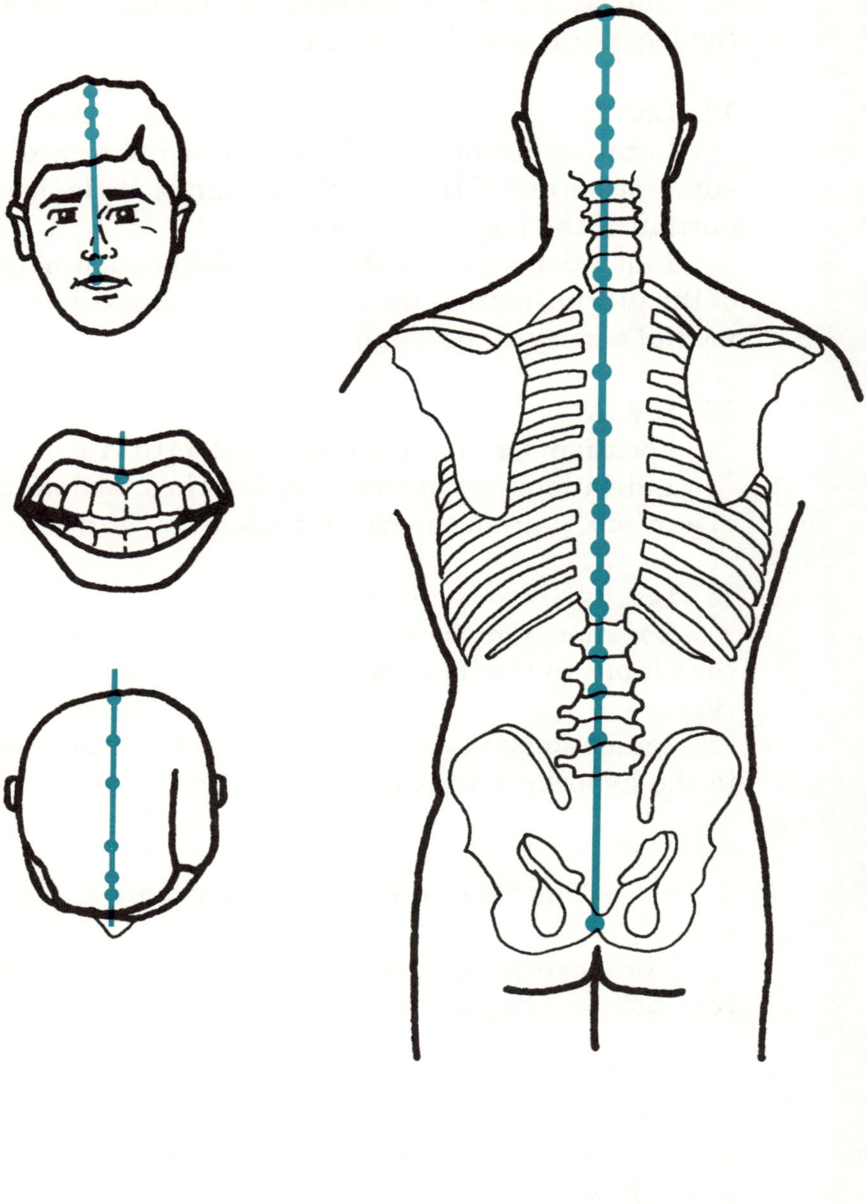

The Governing Vessel Meridian

2. Gv. 2 -

Location: At the junction between the sacrum and the coccyx at the hiatus of the sacrum.

Indications: Pain in the sacro-lumbar region, irregular menstruation, impotence, diarrhea, enteritis.

3. Gv. 3 -

Location: In the interspace of the spinous process between the 4th and 5th lumbar vertebrae. Locate the point with the patient in the prone position.

Indications: Lumbago, impotence.

4. Gv. 4 -

Location: With the patient in the prone position, it is between the spinous process of the 2nd and 3rd lumbar vertebrae, at the midline.

Indications: Lumbago, impotence.

5. Gv. 5 -

Location: Below the spinous process of the 1st lumbar vertebra. Locate the point with the patient in the prone position.

Indications: Lumbago, back pain, enteritis, diarrhea.

6. Gv. 6 -

Location: Below the spinous process of the 11th thoracic vetebra. Locate the point with the patient in the prone position.

Indications: Epilepsy, hemorrhoids with bleeding.

7. Gv. 7 -

Location: With the patient in the prone position, it is below the spinous process of the 10th thoracic vertebra.

Indications: Back pain, anorexia, failing eyesight.

8. Gv. 8 -

Location: Below the spinous process of the 9th thoracic vertebra. Locate the point with the patient in the prone position.

Indications: Back pain, neurasthenia, epilepsy, hysteria.

9. Gv. 9 -

Location: Below the spinous process at the level of the 7th thoracic vertebra, level to the inferior angle of the scapula.

Indications: Cough, dyspnea, jaundice, chest and back pain, stiffness of the spinal column.

10. Gv. 10 -

Location: Below the spinous process of the 6th thoracic vertebra.

Indications: Asthma, bronchitis, lumbago and back pain.

11. Gv. 11 -

Location: Below the spinous process of the 5th thoracic vertebra. Locate the point with the patient in the prone position.

Indications: Poor memory, anxiety, stiffness of back, cough.

12. Gv. 12 -

Location: Below the spinous process of the 3rd thoracic vertebra. Locate with the patient in the prone position.

Indications: Cough, dyspnea, epilepsy, stiffness and pain in the back.

13. Gv. 13 -

Location: Below the spinous process of the 1st thoracic vertebra. Locate with the patient in the prone position.

Indications: Stiffness of back, headache, malaria, febrile diseases, epilepsy.

14. Gv.14 -

Location: Between the 7th cervical vertebra and the spinous process of the 1st thoracic vetebra.

Indications: Fever, heat stroke, malaria, asthma, eczema.

15. Gv. 15 -

Location: At the nape, 0.5 in. above the hairline, between the spinous process of the 1st and 2nd cervical vertebra.

Indications: Deafness and muteness, posterior headache, stiffness of the neck.

16. Gv. 16 -

Location: Directly below the occipital protruberance, in the midline, in a depression 1 in. above the hairline.

Indications: Cold, headache, mental disorders.

17. Gv. 17 -

Location: 1.5 in. above Gv. 16, superior to the occipital protruberance.

Indications: Stiffness and pain in the neck, headache, dizziness.

18. Gv. 18 -

Location: 1.5 in. above Gv. 17, midway between Gv. 16 and Gv. 20.

Indications: Headache, vomiting, dizziness.

19. Gv. 19 -

Location: 1.5 in. anterior to Gv. 18.

Indications: Headaches, dizziness, vertigo.

20. Gv. 20 -

Location: 7 in. above the posterior hairline, midway on a line connecting the apex of both ears.

Indications: epilepsy, headache.

21. Gv. 21 -

Location: 1.5 in. anterior to Gv. 20.

Indications: Vertical headache, dizziness and vertigo, facial swelling, convulsions in children and infants.

22. Gv. 22 -

Location: 3 in. anterior to Gv. 20.

Indications: Headaches, dizziness and vertigo, nasal obstruction, epistaxis, convulsions in children and infants.

23. Gv. 23 -

Location: 1 in. above the middle of the anterior hairline, 4 in. anterior to Gv. 20.

Indications: Headache, eye diseases, rhinitis, nasal obstruction, epistaxis.

24. Gv. 24 -

Location: 0.5 in. above the midpoint of the anterior hairline.

Indications: Frontal headache, dizziness and vertigo, rhinitis, epilepsy, anxiety, insomnia.

25. Gv. 25 -

Location: At the tip of the nose.

Indications: Nasal obstruction, epistaxis, abcess

in the nose, rhinitis, shock.

26. Gv. 26 -
Location: In the midline of the upper and lower two thirds of the upper lip.
Indications: Shock, heat stroke, lumbago, epilepsy, facial paralysis.

27. Gv. 27 -
Location: On the median tubercle of the upper lip, at the junction of the philtrum and the upper lip.
Indications: Toothache, thrush, foul breath.

28. Gv. 28 -
Location: Between the upper lip and upper gum at the labial frenum.
Indications: Pain and swelling of the gum, hemorrhoids.

The Conception Vessel Meridian

The Conception Vessel meridian contains 24 acupuncture points. They are as follows:

1. VC 1 -
Location: In the center of the perineum, between the anus and scrotum in the male and the anus and posterior labial commissure in the female.
Indications: Hemorrhoids, urethritis, pain in the penis, irregular menstruation, prolapse of the uterus.

2. VC 2 -
Location: In the superior border of the pubic symphysis, on the midline of the abdomen. Locate this point in supination.

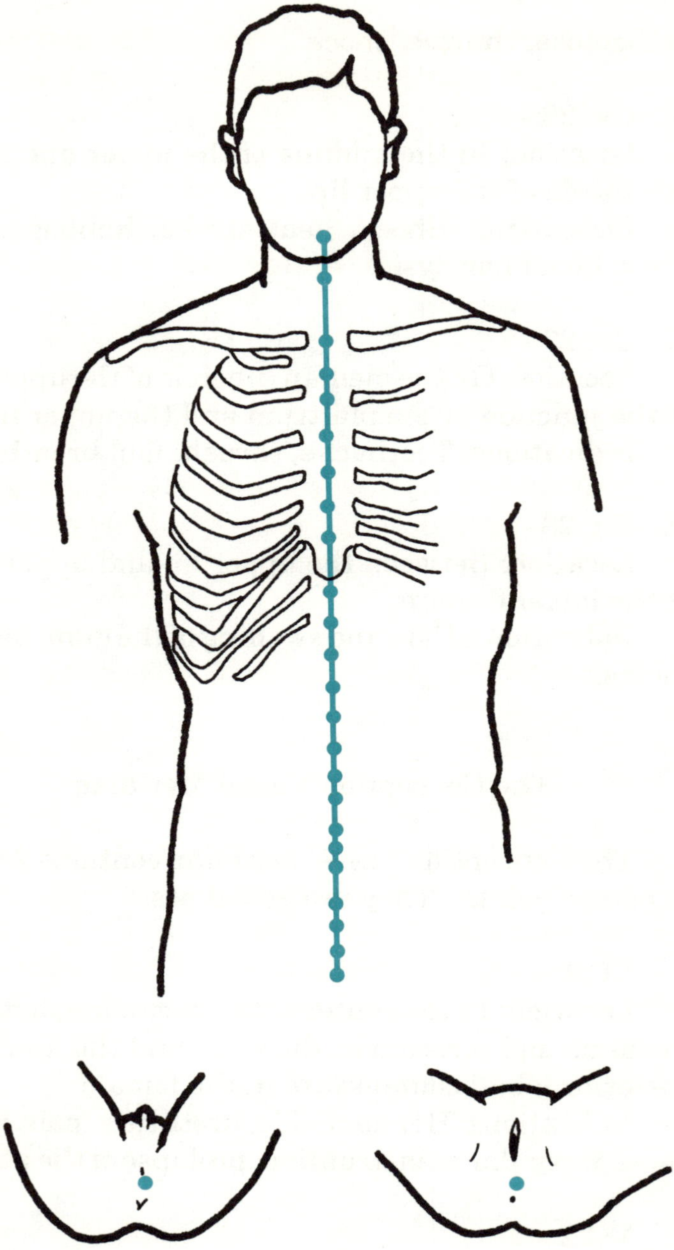

The Conception Vessel Meridian

Indications: Impotence, irregular menstruation, menorrhagia, pelvic inflammation, incontinence or retention of urine.

3. VC 3 -

Location: 4 in. below the umbilicus, on the midline of the abdomen. Locate this point in supination.

Indications: same as VC 2.

4. VC 4 -

Location: 3 in. below the umbilicus, on the midline of the abdomen.

Indications: Impotence, menorrhagia, irregular menstruation, diarrhea, enuresis. This point may also be used for tonic purposes.

5. VC 5 -

Location: 2 in. below the umbilicus, on the midline of the abdomen.

Indications: Abdominal distention, edema, irregular menstruation, amenorrhea, leukorrhea.

6. VC 6 -

Location: 1.5 in. below the umbilicus, on the midline of the abdomen.

Indications: Abdominal distention, abdominal pain, irregular menstruation, uterine bleeding, enuresis, neurasthenia.

7. VC 7 -

Location: 1 in. below the umbilicus, on the midline of the abdomen.

Indications: Urethritis, endometritis, irregular menstruation, postpartum pain, pruritis vulvae, hernia.

8. VC 8 -

Location: In the center of the umbilicus.

Indications: Abdominal pain, diarrhea.

9. VC 9 -

Location: 1 in. above the umbilicus, on the midline of the abdomen.

Indications: Edema, diarrhea.

10. VC 10 -

Location: 2 in. above the umbilicus, on the midline of the abdomen.

Indications: Dyspepsia, gastroptosis, enteritis.

11. VC 11 -

Location: 3 in. above the umbilicus, on the midline of the abdomen.

Indications: Vomiting, dyspepsia, edema, peritonitis.

12. VC 12 -

Location: Midpoint on a line connecting the xyphoid process with umbilicus. Locate this point with patient in the supine position.

Indications: Gastroptosis, vomiting, abdominal distention, dyspepsia.

13. VC 13 -

Location: 5 in. above the umbilicus , on the midline of the abdomen.

Indications: Gastritis, gastric ulcer, vomiting, abdominal distention.

14. VC 14 -

Location: 6 in. above the umbilicus, on the midline of the abdomen.

Indications: Anxiety, palpitation, vomiting.

15. VC 15 -
Location: 7 in. above the umbilicus, on the midline of the stomach.
Indications: Pain in the cardiac region, vomiting, hiccough, epilepsy, mental disorders.

16. VC 16 -
Location: In the midline of the sternum, at the level of the 5th intercostal space.
Indications: Asthma, cough, vomiting.

17. VC 17 -
Location: Midway between the two nipples. Locate this point with the patient in the supine position.
Indications: Bronchitis, bronchial asthma, fullness of chest, hiccough.

18. VC 18 -
Location: On the midline of the abdomen, at the level of the 3rd intercostal space.
Indications: Bronchitis, asthma, pleuritis, vomiting.

19. VC 19 -
Location: On the midline of the abdomen, at the level of the 2nd interspace.
Indications: Bronchitis, pulmonary tuberculosis, pleuritis.

20. VC 20 -
Location: On the midline of the abdomen, at the junction of the sternal manubrium and the body of the sternum.
Indications: Pharyngitis, cough and asthma.

21. VC 21 -

Location: On the midline of the sternum.

Indications: Cough and asthma, pain and swelling of the throat.

22. VC 22 -

Location: At the center of the suprasternal fossaa 0.5 in. above the sternal notch.

Indications: Bronchial asthma, bronchitis, pharyngitis, cough.

23. VC 23 -

Location: In the midline of the neck, midway between the tip of the cricoid cartilage and the border of the mandible.

Indications: Aphasia, pharyngitis, laryngitis.

24. VC 24 -

Location: At the depression in the middle of the mental labial groove.

Indications: Swelling of the gum, toothache, salivation.

14

In applying acupuncture to treat pain, it is necessary to have in mind the distribution of the points as well as the pathological symptoms of the disease. A complete history as well as a physical examination should be done before any treatment is begun. When treating a disease, one should also observe the patient, determine which organ or organs are affected, and analyze the signs and symptoms carefully. Palpation along the lines of the meridians should show which meridians need the treatment and which meridian is the focus of attention before drawing any conclusions as to which meridian should be used for treatment.

The meridians and acupuncture points on that meridian for any specific symptom is not necessarily a set procedure. There should be investigation and collection of data before arriving at any conclusion. Only in this way can progress be made in treating patients with acupuncture. Selection of acupuncture points and formulating a prescription is the key to treating the patient's symptoms. Do not hurry into therapy. Make sure that the complaints are genuine, and that there are signs of discomfort in the area in which the diagnosis is made. Select the points along the meridians, both proximal and distal to the area of discomfort, and select acupuncture points according to the symptoms presented. Many patients will present multiple symptoms. Determine which symptom is primary, and attack that symptom first. A series of five acupuncture treatments are given, using 150 Hz. cycles for 20 minutes, at weekly intervals. Following the series of treatments, a period of two weeks rest is given, and then the patient returns for reevaluation. If the symptoms have not cleared up entirely, then wait two more weeks, at which time further examination is done to see if further treatment is indicated. Then five more treatments are given, repeating the periods of rest and reevaluation.

Examples of selection of points both proximal and distal according to the course of the meridian are as follows:

After determining which meridian is involved select points on the extremity of the affected side below the knee or the elbow. Choose L.I. 4 for facial diseases, TH 5 for diseases around the temporal region, St. 36 for diseases in the upper abdominal region, G.B. 34 for the hypochondriac area, and B. 40 for diseases in the dorso-lumbar area. These acupuncture points are specific for those areas affected. For toothache and mandibular diseases, use St. 6 and St. 7, for eye diseases, use B. 1, for diseases in the pelvic cavity, use B. 32, while for stomach diseases, St. 21 and adjacent acupuncture points may be used.

In the upper extremities, for shoulder joint pain,

use L.I. 15 and S.I. 9. and in the lower extremities use L.I. 11. For pain in the elbow joint, use L.I. 10, L.I. 11 and T,H. 5. When treating pain in the wrist joint, use L.I. 3 and L.I. 4. When treating hip pain, use G.B. 30, and the Bladder points along L. 4 and L. 5, on both sides. St. 35 and G.B. 34 are the acupuncture points of choice when treating pain in the knees. Pain in the ankle joints use St. 41, G.B. 40, and K. 3. Other points can be tested and used if they show improvement in the area.

Pain may be caused when the needle is inserted into the skin, and this should be differentiated from the symptoms the patients present. Most of the discomfort is caused by unskillful manipulation of the needle as the tip enters the skin. Failure to introduce the needle swiftly into the skin can cause pain. Many times, the area in which the needle penetrates may cause pain because of the sensitivity of the area. The direction of the needle may be changed to avoid the sensitive area. It is very important that practice in introducing the needles be performed before attempting the introduction of the needles into the patient.

When the needle enters through the skin into the affected area, pain may be perceived if the needle comes in contact with a nerve, periostium or a tendon in the area. Withdraw the needle slightly and reinsert into an area adjacent to the original penetration. Points located on the face are very sensitive, so it is advisable to try to distract the patient's attention while the needle is being inserted through the skin. Most patients are sensitive to needles, and it is very important that there should be shown concern by the doctor in treating the patient. He should develop their confidence concerning their disease, relieve their anxiety, and gain their cooperation.

The direction that the needle takes after piercing

the skin is very important. When the needle enters the skin, it forms an angle with the skin surface. The degree of the angle depends on the location of the acupuncture point and the disease to be treated. When the needle enters the skin perpendicular (vertical), this method is applicable to locations with thick muscles, or wherever deep puncture is indicated, such as the four extremities, abdomen and lumbar area. When the needle enters the skin and forms a 45 degree angle obliquely with the skin surface, the areas to be treated are the thoracic and back region, close to the viscera and sacral areas. On the face and head where the muscle substance is thin, the needle should enter the skin horizontally, with an angle of about 15 degrees. This should be used in the thoracic area where the possibility of entering the pleura is always present with the resulting pneumothorax on the affected side.

There is no absolute standard depth for needle insertion. It depends on the physical makeup of the individual, as well as the state of the illness at that time. Do not penetrate to a point where damage can be done to the underlying structures, and always use care in inserting the needles. After the needles have been removed, if they are to be sterilized and used again, examine carefully for any barbs, loss of the point of the needle, and straighten out any bent parts on the needle by running it through the thumb nail and the index figer. Most needles that are manufactured today in the United States are disposable needles, and should be used as such and discarded after each use.

The needles may be inserted deep according to the thickness of the muscles. Points may be 0.5-1.5 in. to 2.0 in. in depth. In the lumbo-sacral and abdominal regions, generally a depth of 1.0 to 2.0 in. can be reached on points of these regions, as the muscles there are rather thick. However, the points on the upper abdomen should not be punctured too deeply. The muscles of the back and thoracic region are thin, and there are important viscera such as the heart, lungs, liver and spleen in close vicinity. As has been stated before, the possibility of a pneumothorax by penetration of the needles too deep is always present and should be looked for at all times. It is advisable to puncture superficially mostly in the oblique or horizontal direction. Points along the vertebra and spinal column may be punctured perpendicularly to a depth of about 1.5 to 2.0 inches. On the head and facial regions, the needles should be inserted horizontally as the muscles there are very thin. In order to avoid serious accidents, serious attention should be paid to the depth of insertion when puncturing the points of the opthalmic region as well as that of the neck. The general principle is to master the depth precisely when puncturing points close to important viscera and large arteries. The physician should be familiar with those points in relation to the regional anatomy. Always observe the patient closely when inserting the needles, and withdraw them immediately if any side effects are noted at that time. Manipulate skillfully so as to observe a good therapeutic result and avoid accidents.

Let us review the therapy for the various types of pain, and the location of the acupuncture points for that type of complaint. These points are the ones which I use in therapy, and there are many others that are suggested by the other acupuncturists who practice the art of acupuncture therapy.

ARTHRITIS: Rheumatoid arthritis and osteoarthritis are the most commonly seen in the pain clinic. Rheumatic arthritis is seen in children and young adults. The usual onset is with fever, chills, and aching in the joints. Rheumatoid arthritis occurs mainly in middle aged and older adults. Pathological changes are seen in the joints throughout the entire body, starting generally in the small joints, followed by rheumatoid nodules in the joints of the fingers, symmetrically involved with increasing swelling, pain, and limitation of movement in those joints. In the late stages, there is deformity and the inability to flex or extend the extremities.

OSTEOARTHRITIS is seen in elderly patients usually over the age of 40. Pain is usually felt in the lumbar, cervical, hip, knee and finger joints. The patient aches, and there is stiffness throughout most of the joints of the body. It is a polyarthritis, with aching of the joints, usually relieved throughout the day with movement, but returns at night with immobility and rest.

The acupuncture points to be used in RHEUMATOID ARTHRITIS are as follows: St. 36,37, 39, 40, K. 7, V.C. 2, 10, 22, 23.

The acupuncture points to be used in generalized aching of the joints, with no specific joint being involved are as follows: Sp. 21, P. 6, G.B. 44, Gv. 14, L.I. 15, G.B. 31, 34, 38, 41, B. 60.

LUMBAR PAIN is a common symptom caused by many etiological factors: Sprain of the lumbar region, with no localized pain, and movement of the back is normal. Sacroiliac pain is caused by sudden bending or lifting of heavy objects. There is pain on bending and turning from one side to the other. There is no redness, swelling, muscular atrophy or deformity, except that there is difficulty in straightening the back after bending over.

Other diseases may cause pain in the lumbar region, and may be treated along with the treatment of the symptoms of the disease. Treatment consists of using B. 23, 24, 25, 13, 60, 62, 69. G.B. 25, 30, 34, Gv. 26.

SHOULDER PAIN includes many points of tenderness. There may be cervical myositis, thoracic myositis, tendonitis, bursitis, etc. Pain is felt on lifting the shoulder, movement of the upper arm, and movement of the neck both to the right and to the left. Pain is an early complaint, and treatment must be focused on the general area to get relief. Many times, the pain becomes chronic in nature, and even at rest there is persistent pain in the general area. Acupuncture points which are used are as follows: S.I. 11, L.I. 16, St. 38, B. 57, L.I. 15, S.I. 10. G.B. 34, L.I. 11.

In the elbow, there are other kinds of pain frequently seen other than arthritis. These are (1) Inflammation of the lateral epicondyle of the humerus ("tennis elbow"), and acute lesion of the soft tissue surrounding the elbow (bursitis). Chief symptoms are pain around the elbow, intensified when the arm is rotated in extension. The acupuncture points to be used are as follows: L.I. 11, Lu. 5, L.I. 4, P. 3, L.I. 12, H. 3, 4, LU. 7, S.I. 1,7.

In treating pain the the upper extremities as a whole, use the following acupuncture points: G.B. 11, K. 1, G.B. 23, Liv. 7, 9. St. 31, 34, 36, Sp. 3, 15, St. 32, 37, 39, 40, G.B, 31, 32, 34. L.I. 11, B. 54, G.B. 37, 40, B. 23, Sp. 6, GB. 39.

LOWER EXTREMITY PAIN is usually pain occuring in the muscles both anterior and posterior on the calf. The acupuncture points are different if the knee is the focal point as compared to the foot. For the lower extremities, use the folloing acupuncture points: G.B. 11, K. 1, G.B. 23, Liv. 7, St. 31, 34, 36, Sp. 3, 15, G.B. 31, 32, 34, L.I. 11, B. 54, St. 39. For legs, calf muscles, use G.B. 36, 37, 40, B. 23, Sp. 5. For pain in the knees, use the following acupuncture points: St. 34, Sp. 9, G.B. 34.

TOOTHACHE is most commonly due to inflammation of the dental pulp and around the crown. Select points from the Stomach, Large Intestine, and Kidney Channels. The acupuncture points are:
L.I. 4, St. 44, St. 7, St. 6, B. 23, K. 3.

HEADACHE may be induced by several conditions. Stress and tension are a cause of tension headaches. Headaches may be due to functional conditions, as well as generalized diseases such as hypertension, sinusitis, etc. The following acupuncture points are to be treated for this condition: B. 60, Liv. 2, G.B. 14, L.I. 4, G.B. 20, B. 10, B. 20, B. 10.

TRIGEMINAL NEURALGIA produces pain in the facial area supplied by the trigeminal nerve, which divides into three divisions: the opthalmic, the maxillary, and the mandibular. The clinical feature is the sudden attack of spasmodic electric shock-like severe pain in the involved area lasting from seconds to minutes. Attacks may occur several times a day, generally when the patient is washing the face, brushing the teeth, eating or talking. Pain usually occurs on one side of the face over the area supplied by the second and third branches of the trigeminal nerve. Select the following acupuncture points to treat trigeminal neuralgia: G.B. 14, B. 2, St. 2, 3, L.I. 4, St. 6, 7, K. 24, and St. 44. This is a very persistent disease process and treatment may take an extra long time to get relief.

INTERCOSTAL NEURALGIA is a disease which exhibits frequent pains in one or several intercostal spaces, sometimes with a belt-like distribution. The pain is intensified with coughing, or deep breathing. Select the following acupuncture points: Liv. 14, 3, G.B. 34.

SCIATICA is a common symptom which occurs whenever the sciatic nerve is affected by different etiologic factors. Sciatica presents a diffuse, burning or stabbing pain which follows the course of the sciatic nerve from the gluteal region along the posterior aspect of the leg, the postero-lateral aspect of the leg, down to the lateral aspect of the foot. Intense aggravated pain is felt when walking. The leg stretching and raising test is positive. Acupuncture points that are positive are: B. 54, 25, 57, 37, GB. 30, 34, 39, Lu. 4, 5.

STRAINED NECK is generally due to improper position of the head during sleep, or a slight strain on the neck muscles. The clinical symptoms are usually unilateral pain of the neck and impairment of neck rotation. The acupuncture points that are used for this condition are: G.B. 20, 39, and S.I. 6.

Following childbirth in some women, a condition referred to as coccydynia occurs which is very painful. It is difficult for them to sit down for any period of time. This condition responds to acupuncture therapy, and the acupuncture points that are used are Sp. 9 amd 11. For dysmenorrhea in women, relief can be obtained with acupuncture therapy. The acupuncture points that should be used are as follows: Sp. 1, 2, 6, 13, Liv. 7, 9, B. 23, 47, G.B. 25. For a Sprained ankle use the following acupuncture points: St, 41, G.B. 40, B. 59, St. 41, Sp. 5, K. 3.

15

While practising Anesthesiology at Wesley Medical Center, I was able to organize a pain control clinic in which all therapeutic approaches to pain were used. In treating the patients with both hypnotherapy and acupuncture, I was able to see a large group of patients, whom I followed over a period of three years, sending out a survey every six months to see the results of both hypnotherapy and acupuncture on the relief of pain over an extended period of time. Chronic pain is the number one symptom complex that is being treated by the medical profession today. Many hours of employment are lost due to this problem. Using hypnotherapy, 178 patients with chronic pain were treated. A protocol was set up, and 550 sessions were used for the 178 patients. All of the patients were referred because the usual modalities were not effective.

The patients were given suggestions for the relief

of the pain during three hypnotherapy sessions. During the third and last sessions, a tape recording of the entire session was made, and the patient was instructed to play the tape three times a day for the first two weeks, and then decreasing the number of times the tape was played to twice a week, and then to play the tape once daily after that as long as there was a symptom of pain.

After 6 months there was still about 65% of the patients who were free from pain. After one year 57%, after two years 44%, and after three years 37%. Although comparative studies for this period of time were not found, the results seem favorable for the type of therapy that the patients received. The conditions which were treated were headaches, tic doloreaux, myositis, low back sprain, sacroiliac disease, sciatica, rheumatoid arthritis, and many others. The ratio of male to female was 2:1, with the male patients complaining about low back pain the majority of the time. In female patients, the chief complaint was headache, osteoarthritis, and low back pain.

Beginning in 1983, 378 patients were followed after acupuncture therapy consisting of 5 weekly sessions with reinforcement after three months. The types of pain were similar to those treated with hypnotherapy; however, low back pain was the number one complaint for therapy with acupuncture. After six months, the results were better than those who had hypnotherapy for the relief of their pain, and after one year, over 55% still had relief of their symptoms. After one year, 45% still had relief of their symptoms, and after two years 50% had relief. However after three years, the number of patients who had relief from the pain was 44%, compared to 38% for those who had used hypnotherapy as the treatment of choice. The difference is not significantly different for the two methods of treatment, and the personality of the patient as to the choice of treatment should be a factor at this time.

Many individuals are of the opinion that hypnosis and acupuncture are similar, that there is the use of suggestibility when acupuncture is performed. Hypnotherapy is governed by conditioning. The more that you suggest improvement in symptoms the more you will be successful in removing those complaints. There are no conditioning or suggestions given to the patient who comes to you for acupuncture therapy. Chronic pain is a symptom that needs to be relieved whether or not there is a functional overlay to the condition. The pain is real to the patient, and a method of relief must be found to relieve that symptom of pain. The masking of the symptom by the use of analgetics and narcotics does not help the patient in removing the symptoms. The patient cannot be told, "It's all in your mind, and you must learn to live with it."

In 1958, the American Medical Association approved the use of hypnotherapy by physicians as a therapeutic adjunct within the specific field of their professional competence. There was a resurgence in the practice of hypnotherapy for a few years, and now it is not as popular as it was then. Pain relief, using hypnotherapy, is a part of the practice of those interested in the relief of pain, and is usually included in the services offered by a Pain Control Clinic.

Hippocrates said, "Divine is the task to relieve pain." The complaint of pain is a personal experience to the patient. The physician must believe the complaint, and strive to find a method which will satisfy the patient at that time. Having had numerous types of treatment for the pain, the patient will cooperate in using both hypnotherapy and acupuncture therapy as a treatment for the pain. Rapport between the physician and the patient must be established before either treatment can begin. Understanding the methodology can further help in finding a cure for that patient's symptoms.

What does the future hold for hypnosis? Reading the history of hypnosis, one sees the rising and falling of interest by the professional in using hypnosis for the many symptoms which could be treated by hypnosis. When I started to develop an interest in hypnosis, there were many physicians in my community who thought that there was a future in learning to incorporate hypnotherapy into their practice; however, they soon dropped hypnosis as a part of their practice, since it was time consuming, and the results were not as great as with other therapies which they could use. Will we see another rise in its use in the future? The subject still is not taught at the medical schools as a separate entity, and I doubt whether or not it will be. It is incorporated into the psychiatrist's curiculum, but there is not the emphasis that could be given to the subject.

Hilgard (1983) has stated that "Because of its historical association with magic and mysticism, hypnosis has had to struggle to become disentangled from occult and faith healing methods. The successes of various methods of relieving pain are instructive, but the failures must also be recognized; reliance upon criticized findings is the essence of science."

Today we are looking at hypnosis from another point of view. E. L. Rossi and David B. Cheek have just published MIND-BODY THERAPY: Methods of Ideodynamic healing in Hypnosis (1988). In the Introduction the statement is made as to whether we should still look at healing using hypnotherapy as occurring at the physiological level or whether we should accept the fact that its therapeutic effect is merely the result of suggestion and imagination only. This should create a lot of confusion in the minds of many, but we do know that on certain occasions, the mere use of a suggestion eliminates the discomfort which has been caused by trauma or stress. Much more work will be done in the future on this subject, and we will notice the advancement of hypnotherapy in trying to arrive at a conclusion which will be of sound researchable evidence.

In addition, there is the question that has been raised as to the explanation of the hypnotic state relative to brain dominance, i.e., right brain and left brain. The cerebral hemispheres contain association areas that control abstract thought, logic, emotion and language. The left brain has the function of interpreting content, and the right brain deals with the context. There is also the conscious and the non-dominant or non-conscious brain. When hypnosis is induced into a subject, the possibility of the conscious brain moving off into an area for logical reasoning which then allows the non-dominant or non-conscious to move to the front and accept the cues and suggestions that will be used in the future for relief of symptoms for that subject. In many individuals, we notice that there is freer communication between the conscious and non-conscious mind, and the results are accomplished much more easily than with others. There is still a lot of research to be done in these areas in order to fully understand what we want to do in defining what is meant by a hypnotic state.

BIBLIOGRAPHY

HYPNOSIS

Adams, Paul. THE NEW SELF-HYPNOSIS. North Hollywood, Calif. Wilshire Book Co., 1967.

Cheek, D. B. and LeCron, L. M. CLINICAL HYPNOTHERAPY. New York, Grune and Stratton, 1968.

Covino, N. A. and Warfield, C. A. "Hypnosis and the Management of Pain." Hospital Practice, 20: 48G, 48J, 48L, 1985.

Crasilneck, H.B. and Hall, J.A. CLINICAL HYPNOSIS: PRINCIPLES APPLICATION. New York, Grune and Stratton, 1975.

Deltito, J. A. "Hypnosis in the Treatment of Acute Pain in the Emergency Department Setting." Postgraduate Medical Journal, 60: 263-266, 1984.

Erickson, M. H. "Hypnosis in Painful Terminal Illnesses." American Journal of Clinical Hypnosis, 2: 117-122. 1959.

Guildenberg, P. L. and DeVaul, R. A. "The Chronic Pain Patient. Evaluation and Management." Pain Headache, 7: 1-148, 1985.

Hilgard, E.R. and Hilgard, J.R. HYPNOSIS IN THE RELIEF OF PAIN. Los Altos, Calif. William Kaufman, Inc. 1983.

Kroger, W. S. CLINICAL AND EXPERIMENTAL

HYPNOSIS IN MEDICINE, DENTISTRY, AND PSYCHOLOGY. Philadelphia, J. B. Lippincott, 1963.

Kroger, W.S. "Use of Hypnoanesthesia for Cesarean Section and Hysterectomy." Journal of the American Medical Association, 163: 442-444, 1957.

Marmer, M.J. HYPNOSIS IN ANESTHESIOLOGY. Springfield, Ill. C.C. Thomas, Publisher, 1959.

Melzack, R. and Wall, P.D. "Pain Mechanisms: A New Theory." Science, 150:971-979, 1965.

Melzack, R. and Wall, P.D. "Psychophysiology of Pain." International Anesthesiology Clinics, 8: 3-34, 1968.

Mutter, C. B. and Karnilow, A. "Hypnosis: A Viable Option in Chronic Pain Management." Journal of the Florida Medical Association, 70: 1097-1098, 1983.

Rossi, E. L. MIND-BODY THERAPY. NEW YORK, W.W. Norton, 1988.

Savitz, S. A. "Hypnosis in the Treatment of Chronic Pain." Southern Medical Journal, 76: 319-21, 1983

Spiegel, H. and Spiegel, D. TRANCE AND TREATMENT. New York, Basic Books, 1978.

Tinterow, M. M. "Hypnotherapy for Chronic Pain." Kansas Medicine, 88: 190-192 and 204, 1987.

Tinterow, M. M. "The Use of Hypnoanalgesia in the Relief of Intractable Pain." The American Surgeon, 26: 30-34, 1960.

Tinterow, M. M. " The Use of Hypnotic Anesthesia for Major Surgical Procedures." The American Surgeon, 26: 732-737, 1960.

Tinterow, M. M. FOUNDATIONS OF HYPNOSIS: FROM MESMER TO FREUD. Springfield, Ill. C. C. Thomas, Publishers, 1970.

Tinterow, M. M. and Dicker, M. "Relaxation and Suggestion Training." Physician Assistant, 11: 57-63, 1987.

Wester, W .C. and Smith, A. H. CLINICAL HYPNOSIS: A MULTIDISCIPLINARY APPROACH. Philadelphia, J. B. Lippincott, 1984.

ACUPUNCTURE

Bengston, R. "Physical Measures Useful in Pain Management." International Anesthesiology Clinics, 21: 165-176, 1983.

Brattberg, G. "Acupuncture Therapy for Tennis Elbow." Pain, 16: 285-288, 1983.

Bonica, J. J. "Anesthesiology in the People's Republic of China." Anesthesiology, 40:175-186, 1974.

Bonica, J. J. MANAGEMENT OF PAIN. Philadelphia, Lea and Febiger, 1953.

Collins, V. J. PRINCIPLES OF ANESTHESIOLOGY. Philadelphia, Lea and Febiger, 1966.

Dimond, E. G. "Acupuncture Anesthesia. Western Medicine and Traditional Chinese Medicine." Journal of the American Medical Association, 218: 1558-1563, 1971.

Hansen, P.E., and Hansen, J.H. "Acupuncture Treatment of Chronic Facial Pain—A Controlled Crossover Trial." Headache, 23: 66- 69, 1983.

Huang, H. L. EAR ACUPUNCTURE: A Chinese Medical Report. Emmaus, Penn. Rodale Press, 1974.

Kao, F.F. ACUPUNCTURE THERAPEUTICS. New Haven Conn., Eastern Press, 1973.

Kreitler, S., Kreitler, H. and Carosso, R. "Cognitive Orientation as a Predictor of Pain Relief Following Acupuncture." Pain, 28: 323-324, 1987.

Lawson-Wood, D. and J. ACUPUNCTURE HANDBOOK. Northamptonshire, England, Health Science Press, 1964.

Mann, F. THE TREATMENT OF DISEASE BY ACUPUNCTURE. London, William Heinemann Medical Books, Ltd. 1967.

Mann, F. ATLAS OF ACUPUNCTURE. London, William Heinemann Medical Books, Ltd. 1972.

Melzack, R., and Wall, P.D. "Acupuncture and Transcutaneous Electrical Nerve Stimulation." Postgraduate Medicine, 60:893-896, 1984.

Nozier, P. F. M. TREATISE OF AURICULOTHERAPY. Maissoneuve, France. 1972.

Petrie, J. P. "A Controlled Study of Acupuncture in Neck Pain." British Journal of Rheumatology, 25: 271-275, 1986.

Price, D. D., Rafii, A., Watkins, L. R., and Buckingham, B. " A Psychophysical Analysis of Acupuncture Anangesia." Pain, 19:27- 42, 1984.

Rapkin, A. J. and Kames, L. D. "The Pain Management Approach to Chronic Pelvic Pain." Journal of Reproductive Medicine, 32:323- 327, 1987.

Reston, J. "Now About My Operation in Peking." New York Times, July 25, 1971.

Richardson, P.H. and Vincent, C.A. "Acupuncture for the Treatment of Pain: A Review of Evaluative Research." Pain, 24:15-48, 1986.

Rosen, S. "Acupuncture Anesthesia in the Modern Chinese Operating Room. Personal Observations." In: Risse, G.B. ed. MODERN CHINA AND TRADITIONAL CHINESE MEDICINE. Springfield, Ill., C.C. Thomas, Publisher, 1973.

Van Nghi, N. INTERNATIONAL SYMPOSIUM ON ACUPUNCTURE. St. Petersburg, Fla., St. Petersburg Printing Co. 1973.

Willner, R. E. ACUPUNCTURE DESK REFERENCE. Blackwood, N. J., Ful-Vu Publishing Co.

Yang, Z. L., Cai, T. W., and Wu, J. L. "Psychological Aspects of Components of Pain." Journal of Psychology, 118: 135-146, 1984.

ABOUT THE PUBLISHER

Bio-Communications Press is a service of The Olive W. Garvey Center for the Improvement of Human Functioning, Inc. The Center is a non-profit medical, research and educational organization funded through grants from corporations and foundations and contributions from individuals.

The Center has established three major divisions to carry out its mission of seeking to help stimulate an epidemic of health. These are the ABNA Clinical Services Center, The Bio-Communications Research Institute and The Bio-Medical Synergistics Education Institute.

To learn more about The Center, pictured below, just send your note of request together with a stamped self-addressed #10 envelope to:

The Center
3100 N. Hillside Avenue
Wichita, Kansas 67219 USA

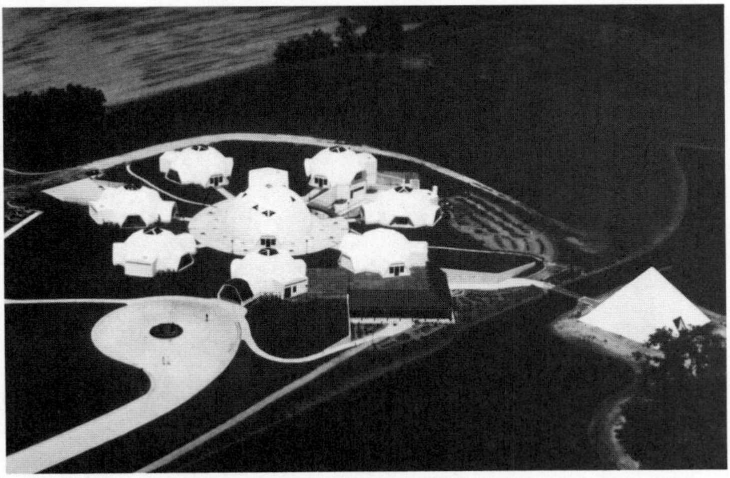

The 21st Century Center Master Facilities of 8 geodesic domes and pyramid

Bio-Communications Press

THERE'S MORE

Bio-Communications Press fulfills a unique niche by publishing fascinating books for select audiences. These books are written by skilled professionals who have demonstrated both a profound interest in their subject matter and the capacity to clearly communicate that interest in an understandable way.

Although our books are not for everyone, we believe what we publish makes a valuable addition to the personal library of anyone who appreciates being well informed on the subject matter they contain.

Our current list of published books:

The Wonderful World Within You–Roger Williams, Ph.D.
The Vitamin C Controversy: Questions and Answers–Emanuel Cheraskin, M.D., D.M.D.
The Schizophrenias: Ours to Conquer–Carl Pfeiffer, Ph.D., M.D.
Medical Mavericks, Volume One–Hugh Riordan, M.D.

Soon to be released:

Medical Mavericks, Volume Two–Hugh Riordan, M.D.
Electrodynamic Man–Leonard Ravitz, M.D.
Health and Happiness–Emanuel Cheraskin, M.D., D.M.D.

To receive a list of books currently available from Bio-Communications Press or to be among the first to know when a new book is about to be released, just return the coupon today.

Bio-Communications Press, 3100 N. Hillside, Wichita, Kansas 67219 U.S.A.

Please send me information about available books.

NAME ______________________________

ADDRESS ______________________________

CITY ______________________________

STATE ______________ ZIP CODE ______________

NOTES